AIDS & HIV

Risky Business

Daniel Jussim

Enslow Publishers, Inc.

44 Fadem Road	PO Box 38
Box 699	Aldershot
Springfield, NJ 07081	Hants GU12 6BP
USA	UK

Library of Congress Cataloging-in-Publication Data

Jussim, Daniel.
    AIDS & HIV: Risky Business / Daniel Jussim
        p. cm. — (Teen Issues)
    Includes bibliographical references and index.
    Summary: Presents the latest facts about the virus that causes AIDS, while also
providing insight on the emotional effects of the disease.
    ISBN 0-89490-917-7
    1. AIDS (Disease)—Juvenile literature. 2. HIV-positive persons—Juvenile
literature. [1. HIV (Viruses) 2. AIDS (Disease)] I. Title. II. Series.
RC607.A26J87   1997
616.97'92—dc20   96-43118
                                                          CIP
                                                           AC

Printed in the United States of America

10 9 8 7 6 5 4 3 2 1

Illustration Credits: Tom Antonie, p. 30; Courtesy of Alex Danford, p. 62;
Courtesy of Kevin Irvine, p. 90.

Cover Illustration: Barbara Bernal Beller

Contents

Acknowledgments 4

1 A Continuing Tragedy 5

2 The Medical Story 19

3 AIDS Comes to School 34

4 AIDS Prevention Programs 48

5 Staying HIV Free 66

6 If You Are at Risk... 85

Where to Find Help 99

Chapter Notes 101

Glossary 107

Index 110

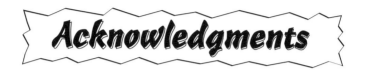

Acknowledgments

I want to thank Dr. Neil R. Kudler, clinical instructor, Department of Medicine, AIDS Program, University of California, San Francisco, for his helpful comments on my manuscript.

Thanks to Alex Danford, Pam Goodlette, Jody Lee Hartley, Kevin Irvine, and Lisa Lynch for agreeing to be interviewed, and for their honesty.

Thanks also to Jenny Jones, M.S.W., and Keith Pollanen for research help, and to Barbara Beller, Leslie Korda, and Andrea Messina.

1

A Continuing Tragedy

———————

☐ Pam Goodlette had her first sexual relationship when she was fifteen. When her parents discovered she had become infected with the AIDS virus, they were shocked—they thought she was a virgin.

☐ At age sixteen, Kevin Irvine found out that he had contracted the AIDS virus from blood products he used to control his hemophilia. For a while, he endangered his sex partners by lying to them and not taking measures to prevent transmission of the virus.

☐ Alex Danford was sexually active, mostly with other males, from age fourteen. He learned that he had the AIDS virus in his early twenties, and is now enrolled in a clinical trial of a vaccine he hopes will help him live longer.

⬚ From age sixteen to nineteen, Lisa Lynch dated a funny bus driver whom she came to love and trust. But he deceived her by not revealing that he was infected with the AIDS virus, and now she is infected too.

⬚ Jody Lee Hartley was infected with the AIDS virus at age fourteen by an older man who sexually abused him. He dropped out of high school two years later, when other students picked on him because of his condition.

The true-life stories of Pam, Kevin, Alex, Lisa, and Jody will be discussed further later in the book. But first we will discuss the history of the disease that changed their lives.

A Short History of AIDS

Scientists believe that the AIDS virus began its life in Africa, where it existed for many years before coming to the United States. The first cases appeared in isolated rural communities in Central Africa. When people in these communities began moving to big cities, they brought the AIDS virus with them and spread it through sexual activity and blood transfusions.

The virus was then carried to Haiti and the United States. It is possible that it was brought here by a group of several thousand Haitians who lived in Africa in the 1970s and then moved to the United States and Europe. Another theory is that gay men from the United States visiting Haiti or Africa on vacation may have brought the virus back home with them.

However it got here, the disease that would come

to be known as AIDS, or acquired immune deficiency syndrome, made its first appearance in the United States in 1981. At that time some gay men began developing unusual illnesses that resulted from a crippling of the immune system. Without their normal immune defenses, they became vulnerable to rare cancers, and their bodies could not fight off horrible infections by germs—viruses, funguses, bacteria—that would pose no problems for others.

Soon, other people—not all men and not necessarily gay—started coming down with the same illnesses: people who injected illegal drugs like heroin and cocaine, hemophiliacs, Haitian immigrants, the sex partners of people in these groups, and the babies of drug-injecting mothers. By the mid-1980s, researchers had discovered the virus that causes AIDS, knew it was deadly, and had pinned down its modes of transmission. Carried in blood, semen, and vaginal fluid, the virus was most often spread through sexual intercourse, the sharing of hypodermic needles by drug users, and, until 1985, blood transfusions.

Some researchers thought a cure for AIDS or a vaccine to prevent it was just a few years away. Sadly, they were mistaken. Also, scientists reasoned that AIDS would spread more slowly if people changed their behavior in certain ways. If they didn't have intercourse, or always used a latex condom (a rubber sheath that covers the penis) during intercourse, and never shared hypodermic needles, the transmission of the AIDS virus could be greatly decreased. This made a lot of sense in theory but was often difficult to put into practice.

One problem was that many people are uncomfortable discussing sex or drug use, and so there was a lot of resistance to frank talk about AIDS in the media; people also resisted the idea of public education programs that would provide explicit information about "safer sex." Another problem is that, for a variety of reasons, people can be very resistant to changing their behavior. The results have been tragic.

The Scope of the Crisis

By the end of 1982, 317 people in the United States had died from AIDS. That, of course, was only the beginning. Through June 1995, there had been 476,899 reported cases of AIDS in the United States— 295,473 people had died from the disease and many thousands more were expected to follow.[1] The disease is now the top killer of men between the ages of twenty-five and forty-four, and the fourth highest killer of women in that age group.[2]

The map on the next page shows the pattern of the AIDS epidemic in the United States. An *epidemic* is a disease outbreak affecting many people in a population. Although the disease has hit big cities on the East and West coasts the hardest, no state in the country has escaped AIDS.

Because AIDS has spread around the world, it is also considered a pandemic, or widely spread disease. While the sexual transmission of AIDS in the United States and Europe has occurred chiefly by men having sex with men (homosexual, or gay, intercourse), in other parts of the world the disease has been spread primarily through men having sex with women (heterosexual, or straight, intercourse). Worldwide, 75 percent of HIV infections have been acquired through heterosexual intercourse.[3] The disease is also far more

AIDS Cases in the U.S.

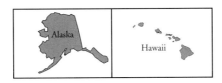

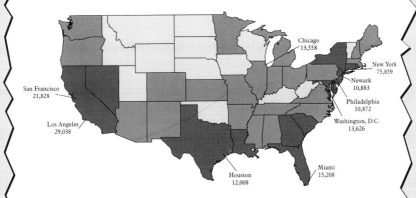

San Francisco
21,828

Los Angeles
29,038

Chicago
13,558

New York
75,859

Newark
10,883

Philadelphia
10,872

Washington, D.C.
13,626

Houston
12,008

Miami
15,208

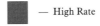 — High Rate

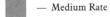 — Medium Rate

— Low Rate

Source: Centers for Disease Control and Prevention, *HIV/AIDS Surveillance Report*, Atlanta, 1995, vol. 7, no. 1, pp. 5–7. AIDS rates are for 1994–1995. Numbers listed for cities are total cumulative AIDS cases reported through June 1995.

widespread in some developing countries than it is in Western industrialized countries. The World Health Organization, a United Nations agency, estimates that 10 million people in Africa and 2.5 million people in Asia have already been infected with the AIDS virus and projects that 20 million Africans and 10 million Asians will have been infected by the end of the decade.[4]

The Victims

In the United States AIDS has been a particularly cruel disease. Because although anyone can get AIDS, it has disproportionately affected communities that have long suffered prejudice and discrimination: homosexual men, racial and ethnic minorities, the poor, and women.

Homosexuals. Being associated with AIDS made homosexuals even more hated by some people. One result was an increase in violent "gay bashing" incidents in the 1980s. Another was the emergence of AIDS activism, as gays organized themselves to fight against discrimination and to demand funding for AIDS research, treatment, and prevention programs.

AIDS has devastated gay neighborhoods in U.S. cities. For decades homosexuals from all over the country flocked to the area around Christopher Street in Greenwich Village, New York City. They formed a lively community based on their sexual preferences and their shared struggle against discrimination. The area is famous for the 1969 Stonewall riot, in which patrons attacked police trying to raid a gay bar, giving birth to the gay liberation movement.

But with a high proportion of gay men in New

York City infected by the AIDS virus, and with thousands already dead from AIDS, the community, in the words of one resident interviewed by *The New York Times*, has been transformed from a culture of "celebration" into a "culture of mourning." This is potently symbolized by a six-story building at the western end of Christopher Street: in the 1960s it housed one of the first gay sex clubs; later a gay bar was located there. But in 1986 it became the site of the nation's first residence for homeless people with AIDS. In the same *Times* article, a forty-three-year-old man who lives there remembered better days:

> I couldn't wait to get on this street because it seemed like everybody was here—black, white, Chinese, Puerto Rican. Everybody was nice to us, whether they were gay or not. You couldn't tell the rich from the poor or the intellectual from the layman. I always made statements to friends that some day I would like to live in the Village, and now here I am, for what it's worth. I got my wish, however it came about.[5]

Researchers fear that San Francisco's gay community, one of the first to be hit by the AIDS epidemic, is suffering a "second wave" of AIDS cases. In 1982, eighteen of every one hundred gay men there became newly infected with the AIDS virus. Thanks to a public education campaign, people learned about safer sex and the community made a dramatic turnaround. By 1985 the rate of new infections had dropped to less than one in one hundred.

But in the 1990s an unexpected thing happened: some gay men started having unprotected intercourse (without using condoms) again, and the infection rate doubled from the 1985 level. For those under age twenty-five, the rate was even higher. A *New York Times* article asked why this happened in a city where almost everyone knows about the consequences of risky sex.[6]

In surveys and interviews people gave a range of explanations that revealed that emotion—not just knowledge—is an important factor in people's decisions about their sexual behavior. For instance, some of them said they engaged in unsafe sex because of depression and despair over the loss of so many friends and loved ones who had died of AIDS. People who are severely depressed don't necessarily care if they live or not.

For some, an intense desire to belong to their community—in which being infected with the AIDS virus is so common—motivated their unsafe behavior. A thirty-two-year-old airline mechanic said, "I thought if I was HIV-positive [infected] I'd be so much gayer."

Others said they took risks because they felt: they had done something wrong, since their friends had died while they survived; sex with a condom was not as pleasurable; practicing safer sex was OK as a temporary measure but not something they could accept having to do for the rest of their lives; or they would become infected no matter what, so why bother to be safe? Some young men believed they would not become infected because somehow they were invulnerable and because "AIDS is the plague of an older generation."

Although AIDS is most concentrated in big cities, the disease is not confined to these places. AIDS is not totally foreign to U.S. suburbs, and even some rural areas are home to people with AIDS. Along with a small town's homey atmosphere, there may be an intolerance to homosexuality that leads gays to leave it for more accepting places like New York or San Francisco. Then, in a cruel irony, in addition to the camaraderie they find in these cities, gay men might find AIDS. Ill, some return to their families in their hometowns. A small town can develop a sizable population of people with AIDS this way.[7]

The Poor and Minorities. As with many other health problems, AIDS has disproportionately hurt the poor. The disease has especially worsened the plight of those trying to survive in America's inner cities. In a landscape where people lead impoverished lives among empty lots and boarded-up buildings, sex and drugs—the main vehicles for spreading AIDS—are among the few pleasures available.

The disease spreads in these places when people who inject drugs share their needles. In addition to the dangers of addiction and overdose, drug users now face the possibility of contracting a deadly disease. The sex partners of male needle users are also at high risk of infection, and when these partners are female, their babies are at risk too. Scientists believe that up to three quarters of all new infections with the AIDS virus are directly or indirectly related to illegal drugs. And, as noted in *New York Newsday*, about 4 percent of all people who use crack cocaine are contracting the AIDS virus each year, "often because they exchange sex for the drug."[8]

Most people who live in inner cities are African American or Hispanic, and poor. Because of their limited political power, the atmosphere of hopelessness, and other factors, fighting AIDS in this environment has been an uphill battle.

New York Times reporter Felicia Lee examined a street in New York City—129th Street between Malcolm X Boulevard and Fifth Avenue in Harlem— as a microcosm of inner-city life in the United States:

> One constant is death, taking the young and old alike. Almost everyone on this block is related to someone who has been shot, is addicted to drugs or dying of AIDS. In the last five months, four young men from the block were shot; three of them died. Here, children talk about the kind of funerals they want in the way that young people in other neighborhoods plan proms.[9]

Early in the epidemic, AIDS was predominantly a disease of gay white men, but that has changed. The majority of cases are now occurring among minority populations, primarily African Americans and Hispanics. This transition is shown by the charts on the next page.

According to a September 1994 report by the federal Centers for Disease Control and Prevention (CDC),[10] allowing for their smaller numbers in the population, African-American women are almost fifteen times more likely than white women to suffer from AIDS; black men are five times more likely than white men to have the disease.

Of minority women with the disease, 47 percent contracted it through injecting drugs, while 37 percent were infected during heterosexual intercourse. African-American and Hispanic men were about equally likely to contract AIDS through injecting drugs (38 percent) and gay sex (39 percent).

Dr. Teresa Diaz, an epidemiologist with the CDC, cited "complex social, economic, and cultural factors"

Number of AIDS Cases Among Different Races/Ethnic Groups

1985

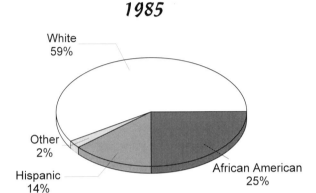

White
59%

Other
2%

Hispanic
14%

African American
25%

1995

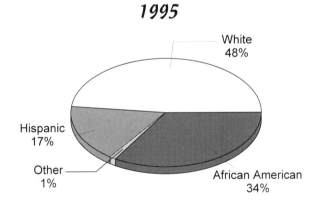

White
48%

Hispanic
17%

Other
1%

African American
34%

Sources: Centers for Disease Control and Prevention, *HIV/AIDS Surveillance Report*, Atlanta, 1995; vol. 7, no. 1, p. 13; and Centers for Disease Control, *AIDS Weekly Surveillance Report*, December 30, 1985.

that can interfere with AIDS prevention among minorities. "If you're poor and live in a high-crime area," she said, "you have other priorities, like violence or crime and other diseases, and may not have such a high priority for . . . AIDS."[11] According to the National Commission on AIDS, which was created by Congress, the disease is closely associated with homelessness.[12] About 15 percent of people without homes are infected with the AIDS virus. Further, between one third and one half of all those with AIDS are homeless or likely to become so, because of sickness, poverty, and a lack of resources. They can be found living on the streets in Los Angeles, New York, Miami, Detroit, and other cities.

Women and Their Children. So far, the disease has affected fewer women than men in the U.S. population, but as the graph below shows, AIDS cases have

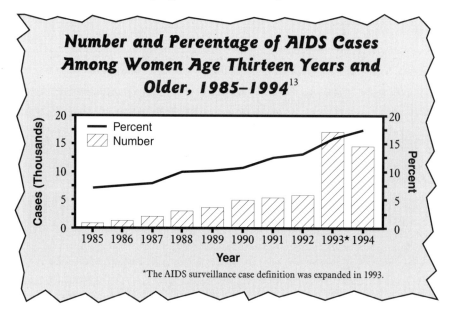

Number and Percentage of AIDS Cases Among Women Age Thirteen Years and Older, 1985–1994[13]

*The AIDS surveillance case definition was expanded in 1993.

been growing at a faster rate among women than among men. While only 7 percent of AIDS cases occurred in women in 1985, women accounted for 17 percent of new cases by 1994. A large majority of women with AIDS are African-American or Hispanic, and growing numbers of women are contracting the AIDS virus through sexual intercourse with infected men.

Some babies of infected women also get AIDS. Out of 4 million annual U.S. births, 1,000 to 2,000 newborns have the AIDS virus. Most women with infected newborns did not know they harbored the virus and could pass it to their babies. But some women who do know deliberately go ahead and have a child in spite of the risks: the chance that the child will be sick, and the possibility that they themselves will not survive long enough to raise the child to adulthood.

Life is so difficult for some of these women that AIDS may not seem like much of a threat. A twenty-two-year-old pregnant woman who lived in a poor community in Brooklyn learned she had the AIDS virus; she was informed that it was likely she would live for only another ten years. Her response? "That's nine more years than I thought I had. I could get hit in the head walking out the door."[14]

One result of parents contracting the disease is an epidemic of AIDS orphans. Experts believe that by the end of the decade, approximately 125,000 children and teenagers in the United States—infected and uninfected—will have lost their mothers, and possibly their fathers also, to AIDS.

The New York *Daily News* reported that some women with AIDS are gathering mementoes to make sure their children have memories of their lives together.[15] Knowing they might not have a long time left to live, these mothers want their kids to have something to reassure them in the future that they were loved.

Among the things parents have assembled in their memory collections are tapes, videos, baby clothes, photographs, letters, and journals. A twenty-seven-year-old mother of a child who is four said, "I've been writing down some of the things we do together—like that on Saturday, we fed the ducks. I have it marked with the date and time we got back."

2

The Medical Story

IDS is caused by a virus. A virus causes infection, and may be thought of as either an extremely simple life form or an extremely complex molecule. In any case, it can reproduce only in the living cells of a plant or animal. The AIDS virus is called HIV for "human immunodeficiency virus." It reproduces in human cells by "tricking" the reproductive machinery of invaded cells—which is supposed to make more cells—into manufacturing more virus instead.

HIV infection does its greatest damage by greatly weakening a crucial part of a person's immune system. The immune system, which is necessary to maintain good health, defends the body against any germs that try to invade it. When you get the flu, for example, your immune system produces special proteins called antibodies, which attack the flu virus. When you feel better again, it is because your immune system has successfully fought off the infection.

But HIV kills key immune cells—white blood cells called T cells—involved in the production of these antibodies. Doctor and writer Abraham Verghese explains T cells this way: "Think of the immune system as an orchestra; it has many instruments, each of which is specialized to do certain things and do them well. When they all work together the body can resist most infections." The T cell "is like the conductor of the immune orchestra." When the T cell is attacked by the AIDS virus, "the orchestra is without a leader. There is total confusion, mayhem, noise. . . ."[1]

When HIV leaves you with few T cells, your body cannot effectively defend itself and you become susceptible to infection. Then germs that would produce no illness, or only a mild illness, in a healthy person can become life threatening to you. HIV is a virus that causes a person's immune system to be deficient. It can also do great damage on its own—for example, by directly attacking brain cells.

Because it can take a long time for the AIDS virus to deplete T cells, a person may be healthy or only mildly ill for years after contracting HIV. During this period the person is infected but does not have AIDS. A person in this condition may not be aware of the infection, and may unknowingly pass the virus on to others.

How the AIDS Virus Is Transmitted

The main routes of HIV transmission are sex and injectable drugs. Neither sex nor drugs, by themselves, *cause* AIDS; rather, they are the pathways on which an infected person can pass the AIDS virus to someone else. The main substances that carry HIV on these pathways are blood, semen, and vaginal fluid. The different ways HIV is spread are discussed below. In Chapters 5 and 6, we will discuss in greater detail how HIV is transmitted through sex and drugs and how to avoid getting it from or giving it to other people.

Men Having Sex With Men. Homosexual men transmit the disease to each other chiefly through unprotected (without a condom) anal intercourse. If one man has the virus, he can pass it to a sex partner when HIV in his semen gets into his partner's body during this act. The risk of HIV transmission is greatly lowered by the use of latex condoms, which act as a barrier to semen and HIV.

Men Having Sex With Women. Unprotected heterosexual sex, although a somewhat less common way to transmit the AIDS virus in the United States, can also spread HIV. Men can pass it to women in their semen, and women can pass it to men in their vaginal fluid.

People Sharing Drug-Injecting Equipment. When people inject drugs, they stick a hypodermic needle into a vein (intravenous injection) or an area just below the skin ("skin popping"). It is a common practice among people who inject drugs like cocaine and heroin to share dirty hypodermic needles. As a result, people inject the blood of their drug-using companions into themselves. If this foreign blood is contaminated with HIV, the virus could enter a needle user's body.

Women With HIV Having Babies. A pregnant woman can transmit HIV to her fetus or newborn. A fetus in the womb shares its mother's blood. If the mother has HIV, her blood may infect the fetus. A baby is also exposed to its mother's vaginal fluid as it passes through the birth canal, and may become infected

AIDS Cases by Type of Exposure

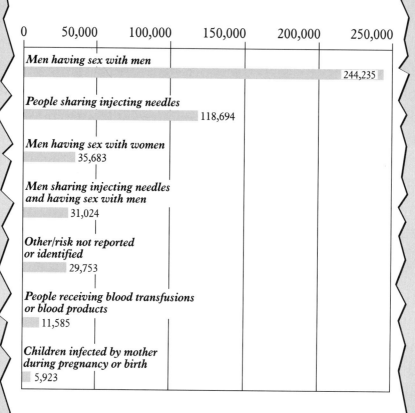

Source: Centers for Disease Control and Prevention, *HIV/AIDS Surveillance Report*, Atlanta, 1995, vol. 7, no. 1, p. 8. The numbers reflect total cumulative AIDS cases reported through June 1995. They do not account for all people infected with HIV, only those among them who have gone on to develop full-blown AIDS.

then. Finally, in rare cases, a baby can become infected through mother's milk, which may contain HIV.

Unless she takes AZT, a drug that helps suppress HIV, a mother with HIV has a 25-percent chance of passing it on to her baby.[2] In most cases of babies becoming infected, at least one parent injected drugs.

Receiving Blood or Blood Products. When people lose a lot of blood, whether through surgery or an accident, they need to have it replaced in order to survive. To meet this need, doctors give them transfusions of blood that has been donated by other people. If the blood is tainted with HIV, they will likely become infected.

Hemophiliacs—people who have a disease that prevents their blood from clotting—use products made from donated blood to help their blood clot. They also risk HIV infection from the donated blood if it is contaminated.

With the discovery of HIV in 1984, it soon became possible to test blood and blood products for contamination. Tests for HIV, which became widely available in 1985, check for antibodies to the virus in the donated blood. If the antibodies are present, it means the virus is too. Tainted blood can be discarded. Blood products used by hemophiliacs can be heated to kill any HIV in them. AIDS transmission through blood transfusion and blood products is now extremely rare. However, before 1985 many people became infected with the AIDS virus through contaminated blood. (HIV testing was also an important breakthrough because it let people know whether they were infected. Those who were "HIV-positive" [infected by the virus] could seek medical help and take steps to avoid passing the virus to people who were "HIV-negative" [uninfected].)

Accidents in a Health Care Setting. Health care

workers such as doctors and nurses may face a small risk of on-the-job HIV infection. Most cases are caused by accidental injury such as a doctor sticking himself or herself with a needle that had been used on an infected patient. Some health care workers have contracted HIV merely by getting infected blood on their skin or mucous membranes, such as their mouth or eyes. The risk is somewhat greater for obstetricians and surgeons. During labor and delivery an obstetrician handles a liter or more of blood and amniotic fluid.

Cases in which people have contracted HIV while visiting doctors or dentists are extremely rare, but they have occurred. In one case, a Florida dentist with AIDS is believed by medical experts to have infected six patients. Investigators don't know how these patients were infected. One possibility is that the dentist accidentally cut himself, and his blood then came into contact with a patient's dental wound. In a 1989 incident in Australia, four patients seeing a surgeon on the same day were infected with HIV from a fifth patient as a result of faulty infection-control procedures.[3]

How the AIDS Virus Is Not Transmitted

Although it can do great harm, the AIDS virus is actually quite weak. It lives in the body, but when exposed to the air it dies in minutes. That makes it hard to become infected accidentally.

The types of HIV transmission discussed so far are basically the only ones known to exist. It is extremely unlikely that you could become infected any other way. Neither mosquitoes nor other insects transmit AIDS. You cannot become infected by donating blood, because the equipment used to draw the blood is used only once. You cannot become infected by casual contact, such as by being in the same room with someone who has the virus, eating at the same table, or using the same computer keyboard or water fountain.

More than twelve rigorous studies have shown that people with HIV do not transmit the virus to others living in the same household—except through sex and shared needles. The federal National Institutes of Health has reported: "Studies of families of H.I.V.-infected people have clearly shown that H.I.V. is not spread through casual contact such as the sharing of food utensils, towels and bedding, swimming pools, telephones or toilet seats."[4]

Freak incidents—rare exceptions that do not affect the general rule—are possible however. In two cases made public in late 1993, HIV may have been spread in unusual ways between two sets of youngsters.[5] Investigators believed that blood was probably the culprit. In one case, an infected teenager may have passed HIV to his teen brother when they shared a razor; in the other, an infected young child had frequent nosebleeds and may have transmitted HIV to another child with dermatitis, a condition that can cause breaks in the skin.

HIV/AIDS Diseases

The first signs of HIV infection often involve health complaints that bother almost everyone from time to time—for instance, diarrhea, swollen glands, fatigue, or headaches. Infected people who experience these maladies and are not aware of having HIV may think they are suffering from the flu or another ordinary infection. Usually, though, such problems are more severe if caused by HIV.

Other frequently occurring early signs include: fevers that are higher than 103 degrees and last for more than three days; severe gum disease; a cough producing phlegm and lasting for weeks; sudden severe weight loss not caused by a diet; not gaining weight, if the person is still growing; a thick whitish coating in the mouth, vagina, or rectum (known as "thrush" and caused by a fungus infection); night sweats; and skin inflammations. All of these signs can also occur late in HIV infection. They range from relatively mild to life threatening.

Note that none of the signs by itself necessarily means a person has HIV. Also, a person can have HIV without having any signs or symptoms. The only way to know for sure that someone is infected is through an HIV test.

Over time, a person with HIV is likely to lose more and more T cells and experience a corresponding increase in severe health problems. He may get one of the life-threatening "AIDS-defining illnesses." These include unusual cancers such as Kaposi's sarcoma (KS), a malignancy of the blood vessels that causes purplish spots to form on the skin.

An *opportunistic infection* is another type of AIDS-defining illness. This is an infection caused by a microbe transmitted separately from HIV. The microbe poses no serious problems to a healthy person, but can become active and cause illness in someone whose immune system is compromised, such as a person with AIDS. The opportunistic infection that causes AIDS-related pneumonia (pneumocystis) is the most common cause of death among people with AIDS.

When someone becomes ill this way, health officials consider the patient to have full-blown AIDS. A new definition of AIDS adopted in 1993 said that even if someone has no illness, that person has AIDS if his or her T cell count drops below 200 (healthy people have T cell counts ranging from 600 to 1200).

In 1996, breakthroughs were made in drug treatments that dramatically improved the outlook for people infected with the AIDS virus. For many of those with access to the new drugs, AIDS may no longer be a death sentence. However, many people will not be able to afford them. Untreated, a person infected with HIV will take an average of about ten years to develop full-blown AIDS, with some people getting AIDS in a year or two and others taking much longer.

Before 1996, only 50 percent of patients were still alive a year after a diagnosis of AIDS; almost none survived five years. Many more HIV-infected individuals do not have AIDS than do have it. Those who receive treatment may put off developing AIDS indefinitely. But it is likely that people without access to new treatments will eventually get AIDS and die.

AIDS and TB

AIDS has helped create a resurgence of the bacterial disease tuberculosis (TB), which had become rare in the United States. Since the late 1980s, the rate of new TB cases has been climbing by 3 to 6 percent per year; health officials reported 21,479 new cases to the U.S. Centers for Disease Control and Prevention (CDC) in 1993.[6]

People with AIDS are vulnerable to TB, which affects the lungs, because of their weak immune systems. Although TB is usually treatable, some deadly new strains of the disease have developed resistance to drugs that used to be effective against it. These new strains often arise when a patient does not complete the treatment, which extends over a long period.

Because tuberculosis can be contagious—you can

Now you can understand what the name AIDS means:

☐ **a**cquired—a person gets it from his or her environment; it does not develop in the body on its own.

☐ **i**mmuno**d**eficiency—it causes the immune system to become deficient.

☐ **s**yndrome—it is not a single disease but a group of diseases.

get it through prolonged exposure to someone with active TB—health care officials have taken strict measures to make sure that patients take all their medicine on schedule. Health workers often ensure compliance by directly watching patients take anti-TB drugs at clinics or at home. In extreme cases, uncooperative patients are confined to hospitals until they complete their treatment, some for more than a year.[7]

The Search for a Cure

When HIV gets into your body, your immune system tries to attack it, as it would any foreign invader. But the AIDS virus is a wily adversary. Its assault on T cells helps disarm the immune response against it, and its ability to mutate, or change form, rapidly makes it difficult for the immune system to recognize the virus and deal with it effectively. This ability has also severely complicated the search for a cure for AIDS. Many attempts to find a cure have ended in disappointment, but new advances have made scientists more optimistic that the disease can eventually be conquered.

Antiviral drugs like AZT (azidothymidine) delay the immune system failure that occurs with AIDS. Eventually, however, HIV mutates until it can get around these drugs. Another problem with the drugs is that they are highly toxic, and can do harm to human cells while attacking the virus.

AZT has been found effective in reducing the transmission of HIV from infected mothers to their newborns. Without treatment, women with HIV pass the virus to their babies in about one out of four cases. AZT decreases the odds that the baby will be infected to one out of twelve.[8] This has created a controversy over whether all pregnant women should be tested for HIV—even those who do not want to be—and whether those who test positive should be forced to take AZT.

A new family of antiviral drugs called "protease inhibitors" is now an important part of the pharmaceutical arsenal deployed in the war against AIDS. In 1996, a medicinal cocktail consisting of a protease inhibitor, AZT, and another powerful drug called 3TC proved effective in fighting HIV in some very ill patients—putting their AIDS into remission and prolonging their lives. Some people who were preparing to die soon—who had put their affairs in order and said good-bye to loved ones—experienced dramatic turnarounds with this new treatment. Suddenly they felt better, and the AIDS virus could not be detected in their bloodstreams. They had been given their lives back. The combination therapy is also being tried with newly infected individuals to see if it can eradicate the virus in their bodies.

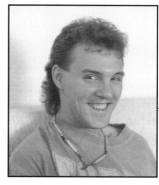

Jody Lee Hartley

Jody Lee Hartley, age twenty-six, was infected with HIV the summer he turned fourteen. An older male co-worker at a small-town Kansas restaurant won his trust and then took terrible advantage of Jody, physically and sexually abusing him. The man also passed the AIDS virus along to his victim. Doctors didn't know too much about AIDS back then, and all they told Jody was that he probably would not live to be eighteen.

Jody says his mother tried to put him into foster care. He then dropped out of high school at age sixteen, when rumors started flying and his peers "picked on me hard."

He did not return to school until age twenty-three, when he trained to be a home health aide in Austin, Texas. He found the work—helping elderly people to dress, clean, shop, eat—rewarding. Unfortunately, although he posed no danger to his charges, he was fired when his employers found out he had HIV. "It wasn't legal," as Jody puts it, "but they told me they had more lawyers and more money than I did, and they could drag out [a lawsuit] so far that I wouldn't live to the court date."

After losing his job—and his home and car—Jody became depressed and attempted suicide, taking 140 sleeping pills. When he survived, he decided there was a reason: He should be doing AIDS education.

Jody now lives in Portland, Maine. As the youngest person in that state to be public about having HIV, Jody spoke to ten thousand young people in more than two hundred programs last year—in spite of the fatigue he suffers from having HIV. Many of them, he says, told him they had experienced some form of sexual abuse and that they had never realized this posed a risk of HIV infection.

Unfortunately, this therapy costs tens of thousands of dollars, and many people with AIDS are poor, with no health insurance. They would not likely be able to afford the treatment.[9] Also, a small minority of patients do not respond to protease inhibitors; others may experience serious side effects, including nausea, diarrhea, and fatigue. Another problem is that over the long term, the drugs could prove toxic.

Researchers are also attacking the AIDS virus at the genetic level. As we discussed, HIV can reproduce only by tricking human immune cells into manufacturing more of the virus. If scientists can alter these cells genetically, it may prevent HIV from using them in this way, leaving the virus to die off.

Finally, scientists have discovered that a small minority of the population is naturally resistant or immune to HIV, and this has given them another important clue into how the virus might be destroyed. To get inside T cells, HIV must hitch a ride on a special protein—called CKR5—that lodges on the surface of these cells. People who have a genetic mutation that causes them not to produce this protein seem to be protected from the AIDS virus. Nobel laureate Dr. David Baltimore sums up the stunning implications of this finding for the rest of the population: "[CKR5] is in fact the key receptor through which people get infected. . . . People can live perfectly well without CKR5. . . . If you can develop a drug that blocks CKR5, it could block H.I.V. without serious side effects."[10]

Of course, a cure would probably not mean the end of AIDS any time soon. The millions of people with AIDS in developing countries do not have enough money to pay for high-tech medicine, and they are not infected with the same strains of HIV that now prey on industrialized countries.

Treating AIDS-Related Diseases

Significant advances have also been made in treating or preventing some of the serious diseases associated with AIDS. For instance, the drug trimethoprimsul-famethoxazole helps prevent AIDS-related pneumonia, increasing people's life expectancy and improving the quality of their lives. Thanks to this and other pneumonia-fighting drugs, people with AIDS live an average of one year longer than they otherwise would.

Unfortunately, virtually all of the drugs used to treat AIDS-related diseases or to fight HIV directly are very expensive. Although programs exist to help those who are poor or do not have health insurance to pay for these drugs, many people still do not have access to all of the medicines available.

Prevention

Some scientists have been trying, so far without success, to develop a vaccine that would prevent people from contracting HIV. According to a *New York Times Magazine* cover story,[11] using a substance called gp120 is the most promising idea yet.

The core of the human immunodeficiency virus is its lethal weapon. There lurks the virus's AIDS-causing genetic instructions (RNA). A protein coat surrounds this core. When isolated from the core, the coat is not dangerous. Gp120 is a copy of a piece of this coat, synthesized in a laboratory. Scientists hope that when this harmless substance is injected into a human's body, the immune system will mistake it for an attack by real HIV. The defensive immune response that results—the production of antibodies to HIV—could then protect a person exposed to the AIDS virus in the future.

But gp120 has run into various problems. It is not nearly 100 percent effective, and no one knows just how effective it would be. Because of this and other problems, experimental trials of gp120 have not gotten past the early stages in the United States. However, the government of Thailand has begun vaccine trials. The results will not be known for a few years.

Until a reliable vaccine is produced, the spread of AIDS can be stopped only by people changing their behavior. This means not having sex, or always using condoms, and not sharing hypodermic needles. Convincing people to change their behavior in these ways, however, has often proved difficult.

For instance, a European study showed that condoms, when used every time people have intercourse, can be highly effective in preventing the transmission of HIV. Unfortunately, it also showed that many people will not use condoms consistently, even when there is a high risk that they will get HIV. For two years, the study followed 256 heterosexual couples in which one partner was HIV-positive and the other HIV-negative.

Although all the couples had been counseled about the risk of infection to the HIV-negative partner—and the protection offered by condoms—121 of them (47 percent) failed to use condoms consistently when they had sexual intercourse. In twelve (10 percent) of these couples, the HIV-negative partner became infected. However, in the couples who did use condoms consistently, not one of the HIV-negative partners became infected.[12]

AIDS prevention through such behavior change is discussed further in Chapters 4 and 5.

3

AIDS Comes to School

The nation's schools have become flash points in the AIDS crisis. Many AIDS prevention programs are held at schools, and the controversies created by them will be discussed in Chapter 4. This chapter covers a different subject: the controversy that arises when students with AIDS want to continue attending school.

Although they may be ill, students with HIV or AIDS may feel well enough to go to class when they do not have symptoms. They want to attend school to learn, to enjoy the company and intellectual stimulation of their friends and teachers, to get out of the house and avoid isolation—to lead as normal a life as possible. This may also help them cope with the potentially devastating emotional consequences of living with a deadly disease.

But their presence in school is sometimes resisted by teachers, other students, and the parents of these students, who may fear that a sick student will accidentally spread AIDS. This chapter will discuss the stories of three teens with AIDS who risked rejection by their communities in order to attend school.

Ryan White

In August 1984, Ryan White of Kokomo, Indiana, entered seventh grade at Western Middle School.[1] He was hospitalized with pneumonia the following December. A hemophiliac, the boy now learned he had contracted HIV from contaminated factor VIII (see box on next page). When Ryan recovered, he felt he was well enough to attend school again, and his mother, Jeanne, agreed.

But the Western School superintendent and the local school board decided to keep Ryan out of school. They feared he could give AIDS to other students or teachers. They argued that Ryan could be barred under a 1949 state law prohibiting children with communicable diseases from attending class.

Ryan was upset with the board's decision. He told his mother, "I want to be with my friends, like everybody else."

National television news programs became interested in Ryan's story, and their interviews with him made his plight widely known. Ryan and his mother were backed up by the state health commissioner and the *Kokomo Tribune,* which wrote editorials supporting him.

Hemophilia and AIDS

Hemophilia is an inherited disease that almost exclusively affects males. The blood of those afflicted does not clot normally because it lacks a protein, usually one called factor VIII, which other people produce naturally. At one time hemophiliacs led difficult lives. They could not participate in activities in which they might be injured because they risked bleeding to death. Often they could not attend school or hold a job. Many became permanently crippled from internal bleeding.

This changed with advances in treating hemophilia, culminating in the development of factor VIII concentrate, which became available in 1970. A hemophiliac can inject this substance when he is injured, or use it preventively. With factor VIII concentrate, he can lead a close-to-normal life.

Factor VIII, though, proved to have a serious drawback. A single dose of it is made with blood drawn from several thousand donors. In a year, a hemophiliac can be exposed to more than a million blood samples. If even a small portion of them is tainted with the AIDS virus, he can contract HIV.

About half of the 20,000 people with hemophilia in the United States are HIV-positive—infected before the blood test for the virus became available in 1985. More than 4,000 hemophiliacs with HIV have developed AIDS—622 of them between thirteen and nineteen years old.[2]

The members of the school administration held to their position. They wanted guarantees that AIDS could not be transmitted casually—or that they would not be legally liable if someone got AIDS from Ryan. But a 100 percent guarantee could not be given. Health officials could say only that the risk of transmitting AIDS by casual contact in school is minuscule—much, much smaller, for example, than the risk of a deadly traffic accident on the way to school.

The community supported the administration's decision. Teachers at the school all agreed not to accept Ryan in their classes. Parents signed petitions backing the board. They planned a lawsuit if Ryan was admitted. And some people went further. According to Ann Marie Cunningham, coauthor with Ryan of his autobiography, "The Whites were generally shunned, even in their Methodist church. The family got nasty anonymous letters, piles of garbage were left on their lawn, and someone even fired a bullet through their front window."[3] Shots were also fired at a *Kokomo Tribune* reporter considered sympathetic to Ryan.

Jeanne White hired an attorney to file a lawsuit of her own. It complained that by keeping Ryan out, the school district was illegally discriminating against a disabled student. Ryan soon became an international celebrity, and could count among his friends superstars like Olympic diving champion Greg Louganis, Elton John, and Michael Jackson. He received letters of support, money, and gifts from all over the world. Still, he said, he would have traded it all in a second to be just a regular kid.

Ryan was in an ironic position—he had lots of support, but little of it came from where he lived. The people in town said it was easy for outsiders to support him; after all, *their* children were not being asked to go to school with Ryan.

In 1986 a court order allowed Ryan to return to school. But this turned out to be a hollow victory. He was not welcomed back but greeted with cruelty and hostility. His classmates stayed away from him and taunted him with jokes, such as: What do gays eat? *Ryan White bread.*

A girlfriend stopped talking to him. Things were stolen from his locker. Eventually Ryan moved with his mother to Cicero, a nearby town. He had become seriously ill again, and, according to *People* magazine, he told his mother he had had enough of Kokomo: "I didn't want to die there. I really didn't want to be buried there."

Over time his condition worsened. By late 1989 he was suffering from shingles (a painful inflammation of nerves caused by the herpes virus), sores that wouldn't heal, and an intensely sore throat. He died in March 1990.

Why the Fear?

Understandably, the parents in Kokomo did not want to expose their children to any risk of disease. But why were they afraid to send their kids to school with Ryan when the risks of HIV transmission were so low? There are several possible answers to this question.

Today, more than fifteen years into the AIDS epidemic, there still has not been a single known case of a student accidentally transmitting HIV at school. But in 1985 the disease had been known to the public for only about four years, and for a while scientists disagreed about how it was spread. People were not as educated about AIDS as they are now.

Author David Kirp believes that parents' fears stemmed partly from a report in the May 1983 issue of the prestigious *Journal of the American Medical Association*.[4] The report said that people could give each other HIV in casual ways, just by living in the same household. This would mean the disease could be transmitted easily—maybe, for example, by sharing a toothbrush or eating utensils. Although the report proved to be wrong, it greatly influenced many people's outlook on AIDS. Some citizens of Kokomo may have believed their children could contract HIV by as simple an act as sharing Ryan's fork at lunchtime.

By late in the controversy over Ryan, scientists nearly all agreed that casual transmission of HIV was not a risk. Studies showed that within the same household—where people have closer contact than at schools—those with HIV do not transmit the virus to others, unless they practice risky behaviors. But people still clung to their fears. This may have been partly due to distrust of scientists. After all, health officials had assured the public that the blood supply was safe from AIDS, and that promise turned out to be tragically false (until the blood test for HIV became available in 1985). Maybe they were wrong about the potential threat posed by kids like Ryan White, too.

Also, people are not always rational, and fear does not necessarily take orders from logic. Consider those who fear flying in commercial airplanes. Statistically, flying is safer than driving; you can tell people this over and over again while their plane is taking off, but it won't slow their heartbeat. They *feel* safer in a car.

The dread of AIDS, sometimes called AFRAIDS

(for "acute fear regarding AIDS"), may make it hard for people to think about it rationally. After all, AIDS makes people vulnerable to unusual, horrible infections, it is deadly, and it has no cure. The very idea of such a disease forces people to confront their own mortality, which can be extremely frightening.

AIDS also carries a social stigma that sets it apart from other deadly diseases like cancer, and this adds to the fear. Some people may be afraid of those with AIDS not only because they are ill, but also because the disease is associated with homosexuals and intravenous drug users—groups that are feared by many.

Some people may even blame those with AIDS for their disease. A nurse from Johnson City, Tennessee, said of a homosexual AIDS patient under her care: "He deserved what he got. It's no one's fault but his. And I don't see why we should have to take care of him."[5]

Someone who contracts HIV in a more "innocent" way may be stigmatized nevertheless, a kind of "guilt by association." For instance, when Ryan White returned to school, classmates tormented him by calling him "fag." This was not only bigoted but inaccurate—he had gotten HIV from blood products. To get AIDS, then, may mean not only to be physically ill but to be socially rejected—and that prospect also could inspire great fear.

Combine all this fear with the intensely protective feelings parents have for their children, and you can understand why the parents in Kokomo acted as they did, even if they acted wrongly.

But people do not always act badly under these circumstances. The following story set in a New England town shows that a more positive outcome is possible when a youngster with AIDS wants to attend school.

Mark Hoyle

Thirteen-year-old Mark Hoyle, from the town of Swansea, Massachusetts, loved baseball, and played in Little League since the age of seven.[6] His skills as a shortstop and pitcher earned him high praise from his coach, and people in town knew him from his ball playing. He was considered shy, smart, and extremely mature.

In the spring of 1985 Mark began experiencing weight loss, high fever, and fatigue, and he was winded after only one inning of baseball. Like Ryan White, he was a hemophiliac. Lab tests showed that he too had contracted HIV through contaminated factor VIII. Mark's mother said, "I was in shock" and that the diagnosis was "as if we were handed a death sentence."

When he was feeling better, Mark wanted to return to school, and his doctor supported him in this. His mother had doubts though, fearing his classmates would "make fun of him and think he's contagious."

Late in the summer of 1985, he was told by school officials that he could continue attending Case Junior High School. The decision would make Swansea the first place in the United States to knowingly allow a youngster with AIDS to attend school.

At first, teachers at the school reacted with alarm. One was concerned that he could contract AIDS from Mark, then transmit it to his baby daughter. But Mark's doctor met with them and calmed their fears. The teachers then answered questions from students concerned about AIDS. When the students learned

the facts—that AIDS was not contagious like the flu—
they became strongly supportive of Mark. A number
went so far as to request being in his classes.

Controversy did arise, though. Many of the parents
had the same doubts as the parents in Kokomo about
the wisdom of letting a child with HIV attend school.
One said, "I was so outraged. God, is the kid drinking
out of my daughter's bubbler [drinking fountain]?"
But those parents opposed to admitting Mark did not
organize an effective opposition. And many parents,
including a woman named Susan Travers, came
together to support the boy with AIDS. Travers, whose
oldest son attended school with Mark, said,
"Everything in life involves a risk. Buses, day care,
everything. What's important is that we have to support each other."

Classmates of Mark, interviewed on television,
expressed their sympathy for him. One said, "It
wouldn't feel right if he were home, if he couldn't
communicate with his friends. He belongs here [at
school]. . . . He has a right to an education just like we
do." Another added, "Think of it like if you were in
his position—how would you feel?"

Mark did return to school. Sadly, in the autumn of
1986 he died from an AIDS-related illness. But this
story does have a partly happy ending. Mark had been
warmly welcomed back to school, where he was considered a hero. At his junior high school graduation,
he received an award for being the student who best
demonstrated the spirit of the school. His fellow students gave him a standing ovation. In Swansea,
knowledge conquered ignorance, and people rose
above their fears to act with compassion.

Years after the incidents at Kokomo and Swansea,

people are more knowledgeable and accepting, and less hysterical, about AIDS. But problems remain for children with HIV/AIDS who attend school. According to an article in *The New York Times*, most parents of school-age children keep the illness a secret from school officials, sometimes not even revealing it to the child.[7] The report said that between 1986 and 1990 parents of only thirty-eight students in New York City—a small fraction of all infected school-age children there—told school officials that their sons or daughters had HIV.

Parents may not tell a school about their child's health because they want the child to be seen as normal. As the *Times* put it, "The rejection, taunting and threats that Ryan endured . . . still haunt the parents of children with acquired immune deficiency syndrome." But if they opt to protect their child by keeping AIDS a secret, they may be putting the youngster at risk in other ways.

When teachers know a child has HIV or AIDS, they can take measures to safeguard the child's health—for instance, by protecting him or her from exposure to sick classmates. The illnesses that commonly make the rounds at school, from colds to the flu to measles, may pose serious threats to children whose immune systems have been weakened by AIDS. If a child's condition is a secret, the teacher won't know to take any special precautions.

Some parents go to a great length to keep their child's AIDS a secret: they don't give the child AZT or other AIDS drugs to take during the school day. Thus, the child's medical treatment may not be as effective as possible.

But to parents who hide their child's HIV status,

Pam Goodlette

Pam Goodlette had her first sexual relationship in 1986, when she was fifteen years old. She was surprised when her boyfriend, a hemophiliac, told her he was going to take an HIV test. "I had seen a supermarket tabloid, and it had a picture of a girl with this wild hair, and she looked like she was ready to charge at somebody. The headline said, 'GIRL WITH AIDS BITES SCHOOLMATE.' That's what went through my mind."

When her boyfriend tested positive, "I cried for him and I cried for me." The couple had not regularly used condoms. Pam says, "It never crossed my mind" that she was at risk. Her father was a minister, and "I was taught you don't have sex until you're married. . . . So I never thought, You need to protect yourself.*"* *She decided to ask her doctor for an HIV test.*

Pam's parents were not aware that she was no longer a virgin. When the doctor informed Pam—the youngest in her family—and her stepmother that the teen had the AIDS virus, "my stepmother's mouth dropped to the floor." The rest of the family was shocked, too. "I was a good girl, and this was the last thing that was supposed to happen to me."

Pam thinks that if a young person with HIV had come to her school and warned the students that they could get it too, she might never have contracted the AIDS virus. That is why she has become an AIDS educator herself.

Since becoming infected, Pam has had a number of boyfriends. She says she always discloses her HIV status before having sex, and always uses condoms with HIV-negative lovers. With one of these lovers the condom broke. Nine months later Pam gave birth to her daughter, Moriah, now fourteen months old and so far HIV-negative.

the trade-offs seem worth it. They fear that people will discriminate against the child, that a school's reaction to a student with AIDS will be, "We're wasting our time on dying children"—as one foster mother of an infected eight-year-old boy told the *Times*. Another mother was wary about disclosing medical information concerning her HIV-positive nine-year-old daughter because she had already seen her shunned:

> Last year my daughter was invited to a birthday party—the whole class went—and this year she wasn't. She's very small for her age, and I don't know if the parents put two and two together. She was very hurt. I can't risk that. She's too young, too naive, to go through it.

One New York City child who did risk being rejected because of his illness was Joey DiPaolo. Fortunately, he did not suffer any terrible consequences from disclosing his condition.

Joey DiPaolo

Joey DiPaolo got AIDS from a transfusion of contaminated blood he received during open-heart surgery when he was four.[8] When he was eleven he almost died of pneumonia. After he recovered, he decided he wanted to be open about his disease, telling his mother, "I didn't do anything wrong; I don't want to hide. I don't want to lie." He told a *New York Times* reporter, "I wanted to tell. I could keep secrets, but not that kind."

And so, when he entered junior high school in Brooklyn, New York, Joey let people know he had AIDS. This scared some of them and made others angry; some parents even organized a boycott of the school. But people accepted Joey after two health specialists came to the school to teach the staff, parents, and students about AIDS. He said of his condition: "It doesn't come up a lot. Some kids once in a while ask, 'So how did you get the virus?' Teachers treat me like a normal kid."

When Joey attended Tottenville High School, which had four thousand students, the principal was faced with a new situation. Although he guessed that some students there carried the AIDS virus, none were so forthright about it—Joey spoke to groups at churches and synagogues about having AIDS. But he was treated like any other student.

One day at Tottenville Joey got into a fight with five boys who did not know about his condition. Because no blood was spilled, the boys had not been put at any risk for infection by the AIDS virus (in any case, the CDC says that it is extremely unlikely that someone could get infected through bites, bloody noses, cuts, or scrapes at school). Joey's mother figured he was just being picked on because of his small size, but she told the principal what had happened, and he told the parents of the other boys.

The result was a plan to have Joey make a video dealing with his disease. It would be screened as part of classroom discussions on AIDS. Joey said, "After my mother talked to the principal, I thought those kids would kick my butt. Instead they came over and were nice as can be."

In November 1993, when he was fourteen, Joey spoke to a crowd of ten thousand people at a "dance-athon" held to raise money for the AIDS advocacy and service group Gay Men's Health Crisis. He gave this advice:

> One: If you know somebody with AIDS, don't be afraid of them. Be a friend. Two: If you don't have AIDS, stay that way. Don't have unprotected sex and don't share needles. Three: If you have AIDS or ever get AIDS, have hope and live one day at a time. . . . I have AIDS and that is how I live. It's hard but it's the only life I know.

4

AIDS Prevention Programs

_____

*W*ith no affordable cure for AIDS guaranteed and an effective vaccine to prevent the spread of the disease years away, the focus is on stopping AIDS by changing people's behavior. Many diseases, such as certain cancers, cannot be prevented. AIDS is not one of them. Anyone with the right knowledge and motivation can avoid contracting HIV and eventually becoming ill. People can change their behavior so that they will remain AIDS free.

It is especially important that teens take measures to protect themselves from AIDS. Because teens are at an age when they might begin to experiment with sex and drugs, many of them risk contracting HIV. According to the federal Centers for Disease Control and Prevention (CDC), an estimated 75 percent of

American teens have had sexual intercourse by the time they finish high school.[1]

Unfortunately, many adolescents are ignorant about sex and its consequences. Edward McCabe, assistant director of adolescent medicine at Staten Island University Hospital, tells a story that clearly illustrates this:

> Not long ago, a 14-year-old girl came to my clinic with delayed menses [a missed period]. I learned that she had been sexually active with the same partner every day for four and a half months—without protection. Her boyfriend told her she was "safe" because "you can't get pregnant the first time."
>
> Without immediately challenging her on this point, I explained that even if it were true [it isn't], there was a difference between the first *time* and the first *person*. Realizing the difference over five very long seconds ("You mean . . . they're not the . . . same?"), she started to cry.[2]

Although more teens who are sexually active use condoms than did so in the past, they are still a minority. In a survey by the CDC, only 45 percent of students said they used condoms the last time they had sex.

The consequences of this can be seen in the high rates of teenage pregnancy as well as the statistics on sexually transmitted diseases (STDs) and the AIDS epidemic. Every year, 3 million teens are infected with an STD such as genital herpes or syphilis.[3] The sores that occur with these diseases make it easier to contract HIV. HIV infection is growing more quickly among adolescents than among other groups, and

AIDS is the seventh leading cause of death among people age fifteen to twenty-four in the United States.[4]

According to Dr. Mark Kaplan, chief of infectious diseases at North Shore University Hospital in Manhasset, New York, "The statistics [warn] us that adolescents are the AIDS epidemic's next hot spot because of their high level of sexual activity and minimal use of precautions against the transmission of HIV."[5]

As of June 1995, a total of 89,477 people age thirteen to twenty-nine had been diagnosed with full-blown AIDS. More than 90 percent of these cases were the result of HIV transmission by sex or by injecting drugs. While only 2,184 of the AIDS cases occurred among thirteen-to-nineteen-year-olds, most of the people who came down with the disease in their twenties had likely been infected as teens (this is explained by the time lag between HIV infection and a diagnosis of full-blown AIDS).[6]

The chart on the next page shows how AIDS has been transmitted among people aged thirteen to twenty-four. A comparison of the charts reveals that females in this age group face a much higher risk of contracting HIV through heterosexual sex than do males. Most heterosexual transmission occurs when a female has sex with a male who injects drugs.

School-Based AIDS Prevention Programs

In an effort to decrease teens' ignorance and reduce their risks, the nation's schools are trying to educate teens in AIDS prevention. Thirty-eight states have laws requiring schools to do this. While people seem to agree on the need for them, school-based AIDS

AIDS Cases Among People Age Thirteen to Twenty-four by Type of Exposure

	0	2,000	4,000	6,000	8,000	10,000

Males

Males having sex with males
9,084

Males sharing injecting needles
1,819

Males sharing injecting needles and having sex with males
1,554

Males receiving blood transfusions or blood products
1,273

Other/risk not reported or identified
814

Heterosexual contact
492

Females

Heterosexual contact
2,490

Females sharing injecting needles
1,473

Other/risk not reported or identified
754

Females receiving blood transfusions or blood products
176

Source: Centers for Disease Control and Prevention, *HIV/AIDS Surveillance Report*, Atlanta, 1995, vol. 7, no. 1, p. 12. The numbers reflect total cumulative AIDS cases reported through June 1995. They do not account for all people infected with HIV, only those among them who have gone on to develop full-blown AIDS.

prevention programs have become the subject of much controversy. The question they raise is: Just how should students be taught to protect themselves?

Abstinence vs. Safer Sex. Teens are most likely to put themselves at risk by their sexual behavior. To guarantee that they will not get AIDS this way, they can decide to be abstinent—to not have sex. If they find this option unacceptable, they can learn "safer sex" practices, such as using condoms, limiting the number of sexual partners they have, and avoiding high-risk partners such as injecting-drug users (see Chapter 5 for a detailed discussion). Sexual intercourse is never 100 percent safe. However, studies show that by consistently practicing safer sex, teens can greatly reduce their risk, although they cannot eliminate it.

Controversies have arisen at the highest levels of government over safer-sex education. Former surgeon general Joycelyn Elders was fired by President Clinton for suggesting that students should be given information about masturbation, a totally safe practice. Most AIDS prevention battles, however, have taken place in the hundreds of school districts that have tried to grapple with this issue.

Should schools emphasize abstinence or safer sex? As part of safer sex programs, is it acceptable to make condoms available free of charge on the school premises to students who request them? How explicit should safer sex education be? Should homosexuality be discussed in class? These are some of the questions that have been debated around the nation.

Conservative religious institutions like the Catholic Church and churches espousing Protestant fundamentalism, as well as groups opposing abortion, have weighed in on the side of abstinence. These groups believe that gay sex and indeed any sex outside of heterosexual marriage is sinful. To them, the best way to stop the spread of AIDS would be for people to abstain from sex until they were married, and then to be completely faithful to their husband or wife. If people did this, they would not need to learn about safer sex because their spouse would not be infected (assuming they did not inject drugs).

Teaching safer sex, they feel, appears to condone sex outside of marriage, and it might even promote premarital sex or gay sex. Encouraging teens to have sex puts them at risk for AIDS, other STDs, and unwanted pregnancies because condoms are not 100 percent effective—sometimes they break or are used incorrectly—and teens often do not use condoms. Just as we do not teach teens how to use illicit drugs safely, conservatives say, we should not teach them how to have sex safely. We should teach them to refrain from having sex until they get married.

More liberal groups—such as educators, AIDS activists, and abortion rights supporters—as well as agencies of the federal government defend programs that promote safer sex. In addition to being more tolerant of sex outside of marriage and of homosexuality, liberals feel that the conservative position is unrealistic. While teen sex should be discouraged, they argue, many teens will have sex regardless of what adults advise them to do. And if they are going to have sex, it will be because of desire or peer pressure or not wanting to be rejected—not because they were exposed to sex education.

Liberals believe that teens who have sex should be helped to reduce their risk of disease and pregnancy: they should receive instruction in safer sex, and condoms and counseling should be available to them. Programs that emphasize abstinence often provide little or no information on safer sex. Liberals acknowledge that condoms do not provide 100 percent protection, but they maintain that teens who use them are at much lower risk. Government health officials support this position. Further, the answer to the problem of sexually active teens not using condoms or using them incorrectly is more education, not less.

State and City Governments Debate Sex Education. In December 1994 the New Jersey Assembly passed legislation requiring that schools teach sexual abstinence as the "only completely reliable means" of preventing unwanted pregnancies, AIDS, and other STDs.[7] None of the legislators opposed teaching abstinence, but they debated where the emphasis should be in sex education.

Opponents, including the New Jersey Education Association, the League of Women Voters, and the National Abortion Rights Action League, feared that the emphasis on abstinence in the bill would result in too little information being given to students who were sexually active. A lack of safer-sex instruction would put them at higher risk of unwanted pregnancy and AIDS infection.

One legislator noted that the New Jersey school district that teaches only abstinence had the highest rate of teenage pregnancy in the state. Assembly member Nia H. Gill said that if the bill became law it would "usurp the power of the local board of education and members of the community who work in conjunction to construct sex education programs to fit the community."

Supporters of the legislation claimed that abstinence programs have proved successful—especially in inner cities—and called it "a common sense bill [that] contains nothing harmful or not in the best interest of students." The chief sponsor of the bill, Assembly member Marion Crecco, said, "What our children really need are strategies to help them remain 100 percent safe from all the fears and concerns of too-early sexual activity." Groups lobbying for passage of the bill included The New Jersey Catholic Conference, New Jersey Right to Life, and the Christian Coalition.

New York City has been the site of intense debate over AIDS education. In 1992 there was a pitched battle over an AIDS guide for elementary school students as well as a clash over a school condom distribution program.

Another controversy arose in late 1994 over an AIDS education guide proposed for students in New York City high schools.[8] Before it could be distributed to schools, the guide had to be reviewed by the Board of Education's twenty-three-member AIDS advisory council. Generally, the conservative majority on the council felt the guide was too liberal, while the liberal minority believed it to be too conservative.

Several council liberals complained that the guide didn't frankly discuss homosexuality and condom use. One of them, Dr. Edward McCabe, said, "Adolescence is a period of great experimentation, and even if students don't identify themselves as gay . . . they are engaged in gay . . . behaviors. They may put themselves at risk for H.I.V., and that needs to be stated in plain language."

Conservatives felt the guide put too *much* emphasis on safer sex. "This type of sex education has been a failure throughout the United States," council member Zelig Friedman said, "and I think it needs some correction. Programs that emphasize safe methods of sex result in higher pregnancy rates and higher rates of sexually transmitted diseases."

The proposed New York City high school AIDS guide suggests things to say when you want to refuse sex. Possibilities include:

☐ Let's go to a movie.

☐ Let's invite people over for a party.

☐ My family will kill me.

☐ I don't know you well enough.

☐ If you cared, you'd wait.

☐ It's against my religion.

Studies. Studies carried out on school-based AIDS prevention programs have shown that it is easier to increase students' knowledge about the disease than to change their behavior. Students in most of these programs come away with a greater understanding of HIV transmission but do not act on it by adopting safer sex or practicing abstinence. However, some programs have made a difference in behavior. We will look at one that focused exclusively on abstinence, and one that encouraged safer sex practices.

A program created at Grady Memorial Hospital in Atlanta, Georgia, was designed to help boys and girls resist pressures to have sex.[9] Its first target was eighth-grade minority students at high risk for pregnancy and STDs. According to an article in *The Atlantic Monthly*, the program, given over five class periods, offers more than a "Just say no" message:

> It reinforces the message by having young people practice the desired behavior. The classes are led by popular older teenagers who teach middle-schoolers how to reject sexual advances and refuse sexual intercourse. The eighth-graders perform skits in which they practice refusals. Some of them take the part of "angel on my shoulder," intervening if the sexually beleaguered student runs out of ideas. Boys practice resisting pressure from other boys.

At the end of ninth grade, researchers compared the students who had taken the program with others who had not. While 39 percent of those who were not in the program had had sexual intercourse, only 24 percent of students who had taken the program had done so. The author of the *Atlantic* article concluded, "Studies of similar programs show similar results: abstinence messages can help students put off sex."

An experimental program begun in New York City in 1991 also succeeded somewhat in altering teens' behavior. In this program, New York City students aged twelve to twenty, 72 percent of them African American or Hispanic, received a special six-lesson AIDS prevention curriculum.[10] They were taught the facts about HIV transmission and safer sex; were helped, through discussions, "to clarify their personal values pertaining to involvement in sexual intercourse"; and learned, through role playing, the negotiation skills needed to refuse sex or to use condoms. They also learned how to get condoms and use them correctly.

The adolescents who completed the program subsequently had a decreased number of sexual partners, a decrease in sexual intercourse with high-risk partners (such as injecting-drug users), and an increase in consistent use of condoms. However, there was no effect on their practice of abstinence. While the changes were modest, the program was brief.

In its use of role playing and discussions of values, this program went beyond just giving students information. Perhaps that partly accounted for its success. Many experts believe that while AIDS education is important, preventing risky behavior takes more than giving people knowledge. Behavior that can lead to AIDS transmission is like smoking or drug or alcohol abuse: people know it is dangerous, but many do it anyway.

Because people do not always act rationally, AIDS prevention efforts based solely on education may fall short. Emotion and other irrational factors must be taken into account. As one AIDS activist put it, "It's not enough to tell a guy to put on a condom. You have to make him want to put it on."[11]

Peer AIDS Education. Another strategy used in AIDS prevention is peer AIDS education, in which teens teach other teens about the disease. A two-day pilot program promoting this concept took place in March 1994 at North Shore University Hospital in suburban Manhasset, New York.[12] Teens from a cross section of the student population were trained to be peer educators.

The students received information on AIDS; HIV

transmission; prevention methods, including the use of condoms; sexuality; decision making; and negotiation. They learned about the physical, emotional, and social effects of AIDS directly from people who had the disease. The hope was that they would be able to take this information and spread it to their friends and classmates.

Dr. Victor Fornari, the assistant chairman for child and adolescent psychiatry at the hospital, said that peer programs are effective because teens are likely to listen seriously to other teens. He noted that because adolescents are often rebellious by nature, they may defy adults and any advice they provide.

The National Commission on AIDS, a body created by the federal government to study and make recommendations concerning the disease, found peer education to be "promising," but only when combined with other components of a prevention program. Testifying before the commission, New York City public high school student Kate Barnhart said,

> The peer education approach has many benefits. Peer educators are constantly available. We can be approached informally in the halls, gym, cafeteria, or anywhere. . . . We can be telephoned at home if questions arise. We are not confined to the role of educator or authority. We make the transition to friend easily.[13]

The trainees at North Shore's program seemed to take their role seriously. One of them, tenth grader D. J. Goldman, said, "People think it can't happen to us. We've got to get it across to our friends that yes, it really can happen to us."[14]

Condom Availability Programs. Many city high schools, as part of AIDS prevention efforts, provide condoms to students who request them. New York City has a program in which students can go to special rooms in their high school and receive condoms, instruction on using them correctly, information about AIDS, and counseling and referral services.

This program, copied by many schools across the country, faced a legal challenge from people who felt it violated the parents' right to bring up their children as they see fit.[15] In December 1993 a state appellate court agreed with them, ruling against the program because it did not require parental consent—students were free to get condoms without their parents' permission.

The court majority said that schools could fight AIDS without violating parents' rights. "We must take great care not to be blinded by the concept that the end justifies the means," declared Justice Vincent Pizzuto. The dissenting judges dismissed this argument, asserting that the consequences of contracting AIDS were grave and "outweigh the minimal intrusion into the parent-child relationship."

In the wake of the court ruling, the New York City Board of Education altered the condom program to meet the court's objections: it devised a plan that allows parents to "opt out" of the program by barring their children from participation. Critics said that the new policy compromised students' confidentiality—school officials would have to check the names of those seeking condoms to make sure their parents did not object—and worried this would discourage them from seeking the service. Edward McCabe said in May 1994 that fewer than one percent of parents had opted out.[16]

Other AIDS Prevention Programs

Support Groups. AIDS prevention programs are also offered outside of schools, especially to populations at high risk for contracting the disease. The New York organization Gay Men's Health Crisis (GMHC), for instance, runs small support groups for HIV-negative gay men. In these groups, participants discuss their feelings about sex, drugs, and AIDS.

Richard Elovich, director of GMHC's substance use counseling and education department, said that "sharing deeply personal experiences and feelings about being gay, having sex, and being HIV-negative might lead to increased self-esteem and create some solace from the despair that may be leading them to put themselves at risk."[17]

The subject of drugs is important in these groups because drug or alcohol use can lead people into risky sex by lowering their defenses. They might know better, but that knowledge does not necessarily count for much when they are high. In the words of one campaign promoting safer sex: "Get drunk, get stupid, get AIDS." And, of course, drugs are a vital issue because sharing drug-injecting needles can easily transmit HIV. To combat this hazard, some cities are offering needle exchange programs.

Needle Exchange Programs. Drug addicts may share needles as an act of camaraderie with companion users. Also, because it is illegal in some places to buy hypodermic needles from a pharmacy without a prescription, drug users may borrow needles from friends, or purchase or rent them from street dealers. Often these needles have been used and not adequately cleaned; they may still be tainted with HIV.

Of course, the most desirable way to stop virus

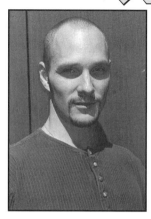

Alex Danford

In November 1994 Alex Danford received a surprising phone call. Would he like to meet President Clinton in the Oval Office in two days? Alex, age twenty-five, flew to the capital, one of six HIV-positive young people who met with Clinton to discuss the AIDS epidemic. "I think he wanted to put a face on HIV in young people," Alex says.

About two years ago Alex moved from his hometown of Seattle to Dayton, Ohio. Just before moving, he had an HIV test as part of a routine physical exam. Two days after arriving, he got the bad news: his test was positive. His reaction? "I lay on the couch for three months and watched American Movie Classics."

Alex had been sexually active, mostly with males, since age fourteen. He knew about AIDS as a teen, and felt it was inevitable that he would become infected. He would use condoms, but not consistently until he was older. "I didn't have the skills," he says. "I didn't know how to tell someone what I thought should happen."

Eventually Alex pulled himself together. He went on to earn an AmeriCorps-sponsored job doing AIDS education with the Red Cross, to co-write a report on young people and HIV for the Office of National AIDS policy, and to become a charter member of the National Association of Positive Youth, which links young people with HIV all over the country.

Alex, who is in good health, is also enrolled in a clinical trial of a vaccine made with genetically altered live HIV. Scientists hope it will train his immune system to recognize the virus so that it can kill it off more readily. He says he is "hopeful that there are ways to live with HIV. . . . Man, I want to live so badly."

transmission by this route would be for people to stop injecting drugs. But injecting-drug use is a problem that has existed for a long time, and it is not likely to vanish because of AIDS. The shortage of openings in drug rehabilitation programs and the expense of such programs does not help.

Given these realities, another possible way to stop drug-related HIV transmission would be to provide users with clean needles and educate them about not sharing.[18] Experimental programs designed to do just that exist in New York City, Los Angeles, Chicago, Canada, and several places in Europe. Usually the programs provide people with free, clean needles in exchange for used ones.

Clean-needle programs are illegal in some states. The controversy surrounding them stems partly from the fear that they will increase illegal drug use or send the message to people that drug use is acceptable. Some African-American clergymen have complained that the priorities are wrong—that the government should provide treatment for people who abuse drugs before it spends money on needle exchanges.

But studies indicating that needle exchange programs slow the spread of the AIDS virus are making them less controversial. A study in New York City—which has two hundred thousand people addicted to injection drugs, half of whom are thought be infected with HIV—supports the promise of needle exchange.

The study looked at a sample of the more than twenty-six thousand people who participate in the city's needle exchange programs, which are run by community groups. Early findings in the study showed that those in the programs have a much lower rate of HIV infection (1 to 2 percent per year) than other New Yorkers who inject drugs (4 to 5 percent per year).

In addition, the concerns that people would increase their drug use because of the needle exchanges—or that nonusers would start shooting up—were not supported. The researchers concluded that clean-needle programs could cut HIV transmission among addicts in half. In an editorial, *The New York Times* argued that if these early findings were confirmed, other states should embrace needle exchange.[19]

But not everyone is persuaded. In Los Angeles members of several Hollywood neighborhood groups engaged in a citizens arrest of people operating a needle exchange program. Mayor Richard Riordan had declared a state of emergency one week before to allow needle exchanges to go forward. He told police not to enforce laws that would stop them, because of all the groups at risk, AIDS was spreading fastest among injection-drug users. But the Hollywood residents said the program was attracting undesirable people.[20]

Similarly, a member of a community board on New York's Lower East Side complained that a needle exchange program in operation there was ruining her neighborhood.[21] She said the program attracted addicts who committed crimes and left dirty syringes in the streets. "Statistics on the spread of AIDS cannot be the only criteria for measuring the success of the program," she argued.

The Outlook

Unfortunately, attempts to improve prevention programs have been hampered by a lack of money and by short shrift given to gays by legislatures. In

California, where homosexual men make up 80 percent of all people with AIDS, less than 10 percent of AIDS prevention funds are targeted at this population, said Patricia Franks of the Institute for Health Policy Studies at the University of California.[22]

Prevention efforts have also been slowed by the federal government's reluctance to pay for studies involving sexuality and drug use.[23] In July 1994 a committee of the National Academy of Sciences said that more research, including a comprehensive national survey of people's sexual practices and drug use, was needed to further AIDS prevention. Funding for studies like this was blocked by conservatives during the Reagan and Bush administrations and has not been revived under President Clinton.

5

Staying HIV Free

---

*T*he bad news is that anyone can get AIDS: rich or poor, smart or not, male or female, young or old, fat or thin, gay or straight, black or white—or of any other racial or ethnic background. The good news is that everyone can make decisions and take actions to avoid getting AIDS.

How You Get HIV from Sex
The AIDS virus can be transmitted during anal, vaginal, or oral intercourse. It can be transmitted from a male to a female or from a female to a male (heterosexual intercourse) or from a male to a male (homosexual intercourse). In rare cases it is transmitted from a female to a female.

The virus is most easily transmitted during anal intercourse, in which a man inserts his penis into his partner's rectum (via the anus). If the man has HIV, when he ejaculates semen, or "comes," into his partner's rectum, the virus may enter the partner's bloodstream through small tears formed in the rectum by the action of anal sex. (Pre-ejaculatory fluid, which is secreted from the penis before semen is released, may also carry HIV.) Anal intercourse without a condom is the single most risky sex act, and the greatest risk during this act is to the receptive partner, the person whose body is penetrated.

During vaginal intercourse, a man inserts his penis into a woman's vagina. HIV in pre-ejaculatory fluid or in his ejaculated semen can infect the woman, while HIV in a woman's vaginal fluid can infect the man.

While not as risky as vaginal or anal intercourse, oral sex—which involves contact between one person's mouth and another's penis, vagina, or anus—may also transmit HIV.

Sexually transmitted diseases (STDs) besides AIDS—such as syphilis, gonorrhea, and herpes—can also be transmitted by anal, vaginal, or oral intercourse. These diseases increase the risk of HIV transmission because they cause open sores to form on the mouth, anus, or genitals. HIV can pass easily through these sores.

Protecting Yourself

Abstinence. The only way to be 100 percent certain not to get HIV from sex is to abstain from having sex. For teens, abstaining has many advantages. In addition to avoiding HIV, you prevent other STDs (every eleven seconds, a teen in the United States contracts an STD). You also avoid unwanted pregnancy (every thirty seconds, a teen in the United States becomes pregnant). By waiting until you are older, you can delay sex until you are emotionally ready for a sexual relationship. When you are more mature, you will have better judgment and will be able to communicate more effectively with a partner about safer sex practices and about sex in general.

It may seem difficult to abstain when powerful forces are pushing you toward having sex. Your instincts and your hormones may make you crave sexual release. Meanwhile, messages from television, movies, and advertising that glamorize sex may lead you to feel you can't do without it. Also, you may want to have sex because your friends are doing it, or to avoid rejection by a boyfriend or girlfriend.

But in the face of all these pressures, you might ask yourself if sex—sex right now—is worth dying for, because that is the risk you might be taking. If you have not had sex yet, it makes a lot of sense to continue not having sex. Once a teen has had sex, he or she is less likely to become abstinent again. And as with condom use (discussed below), abstinence must be consistent to be effective.

It may be difficult to refuse when someone is trying to persuade you to have sex. One way to avoid being pressured is to avoid going anywhere alone with a person who you think might do this. If someone does pressure you, you can tell him or her that you don't want to have sex. Or you can just walk away. When you will be too far from home to walk back, carry change so you can make a call from a public telephone and get a ride from a friend or family member. Remember that no one has the right to force you to have sexual intercourse or do anything else you do not want to do.

Your Right to Refuse

You might want to practice refusing sex by rehearsing what you would want to say if someone was pressuring you. You can use the suggestions below (offered by the Centers for Disease Control), or think up some of your own:

☐ "I am just not ready for it yet."

☐ "I know it feels right for you and I care about you. But I'm not going to do it until I'm sure it's the right thing for me to do."

☐ "I care about you but I don't want the responsibility that comes with sex."

☐ "I think sex outside of marriage is wrong."

☐ "I feel good about not having sex until I'm married. I've made my decision and I feel comfortable with it."

If you are abstinent "most of the time," don't assume you are out of danger. Even if you have sex only occasionally, you may still be putting yourself at risk. It is possible to contract HIV from a single sexual encounter. If you are going to have sex—*at all*—it is crucial that you learn about the safer sex techniques, which will be discussed next.

Sex Without Intercourse. If you want to have sex, you can still choose not to have intercourse. There are other ways to give and receive sexual pleasure and to express affection that involve little or no risk. For instance, self-masturbation is a completely safe act that allows you to learn about your sexuality and achieve release without the pressure of a partner's presence. The physical sensations you experience during masturbation are similar to those of sex with another person—and sometimes even more pleasurable!

If you have a partner, you need not have intercourse in order to enjoy touching each other. Scientists believe that deep or "French" kissing is virtually risk free. There has been no known instance of HIV transmission by this route. Concentrations of HIV in the saliva of an infected person are probably too low to transmit the virus to his or her partner. However, if a person with HIV has blood in his or her mouth—for instance, because of gum disease—it may be possible for the person to infect a partner during deep tongue-kissing, especially if the partner's mouth has cuts or sores in it.

Petting, full-body massage, and mutual masturbation are also safe acts, provided that there are no cuts, sores, or bleeding in the places being touched or on the hands doing the touching. Kissing and licking the outside parts of the body—not including oral sex—is perfectly safe too; again, there should be no openings in the mouth or on the skin.

The most significant risk involved in sexual touching, sometimes called "outercourse," may be that it makes you want to do more—to "go all the way." If you become sexually aroused, it might affect your judgment and make it difficult to stick to a plan not to have intercourse. So you should consider carefully how far

Lisa Lynch

Lisa Lynch of Brooklyn, New York, dated Thomas (not his real name), an older man, from the time she was sixteen years old to the time she was nineteen. She describes the man, who used to drive a bus, as "a wonderful conversationalist with a sense of humor." Soon after they were engaged, he was hospitalized—for kidney failure, or so Lisa was told. He was in and out of the hospital for about six months, and then one morning he died.

The day she buried him, someone in his family came up to Lisa and said that it was not kidney failure that had killed her fiancé. Thomas had actually died from AIDS. At first Lisa did not believe this, but soon afterward she paid a visit to her doctor and learned two more shocking facts: she herself was now infected with the AIDS virus . . . and she was pregnant.

Lisa had apparently been infected by Thomas during unprotected sexual intercourse. They had used condoms, which can protect against sexual transmission of the AIDS virus, at the beginning of their relationship. However, according to Lisa, "In a few months a relationship can build to a point where you say, 'I really do trust this man.' And he looked fine so I wasn't worried." They stopped using condoms.

Lisa's trust was betrayed. Thomas deceived her, never revealing that he carried the virus and then lying about why he was sick. For a while, she says, "I wanted to spit on his grave." But she couldn't hate him "because I was totally in love with the man."

Lisa is now twenty. An African American, she does AIDS peer counseling for the group Stand Up Harlem. Her son is eight months old. So far she has not suffered any health problems from the AIDS virus—but it could turn deadly anytime, and as Lisa says, "It doesn't go away."

you want to go, and you may want to stop what you are doing if you feel your resolve weakening.

Using Condoms. If you are going to have sexual intercourse, protect yourself by using a latex condom—a thin, flexible, rubber tube rolled down over the penis before intercourse. Condoms can be purchased easily at drugstores; you do not need a prescription, and you can buy them at any age. You may be able to get condoms for free through your school, a local Planned Parenthood clinic, or an AIDS information organization.

Latex condoms have been shown to prevent infection from HIV, other STDs, and pregnancy. Studies of couples in which one partner is HIV-positive and the other HIV-negative clearly illustrate that condoms can be highly effective at disease prevention. They also prove that to be effective, condoms must be used consistently—which means every time you have intercourse. Failing to use condoms, and use them every time, is playing Russian roulette.

Sex with a condom is called "safer sex" because it is a lot less dangerous than sex without one. However, because condoms may break or slip off, even correct and consistent use does not make sex risk free. Follow the instructions discussed on pages 74–75, and note that when condoms fail it is usually because they have been used improperly—not because they are of poor quality.

Both partners should be equally responsible for making sure a condom is used every time. Don't leave a decision to use condoms up to your lover. You should always carry condoms or have them available if you plan to have intercourse.

Discuss using condoms with your partner ahead of time in a neutral setting, not in the bedroom or in the middle of foreplay. You may find it difficult and ineffective to interrupt a passionate embrace to bring up the subject. Putting on a condom need not be unromantic or awkward. If you and your partner can think of it as just another part of sex, it can even be fun, affectionate, or passionate. If you want your condoms to look less like medical devices and more like toys, buy colored ones (you can match your socks).

You can practice ahead of time if you have not used a condom before. A boy can rehearse opening a condom package and putting the condom on his erect penis. A girl can put a condom on a finger or a banana. Lovers can also practice together until they can handle condoms with ease.

Two types of condom made out of polyurethane are now available in the United States, and may provide people with new options in preventing HIV transmission. While polyurethane has been shown in the laboratory to block the passage of HIV, further clinical testing is needed to see how well it works in a real-life situation. Because of this, latex condoms are still preferred.

The new condoms come in "his or her" varieties. The female condom, or vaginal pouch, is a lubricated polyurethane sheath held together by two rings, one that goes into the vagina and another that stays outside the body. It is inserted like a diaphragm. The female condom offers some distinct advantages: it can be inserted well before intercourse; and in cases when a man will not readily use a condom, it lets women take their own precautions against HIV. However, some people do not like its appearance.

The other polyurethane condom is made for men, and goes over the penis. In addition to providing an

How to Practice Safer Sex

☐ Use a latex condom with a lubricant that contains nonoxynol-9 every time you have anal or vaginal intercourse. For oral sex, use an unlubricated condom.

☐ Latex serves as a barrier to the AIDS virus. Lambskin or natural-membrane condoms have pores (tiny holes) in the material that permit transmission of HIV and other STDs. Look for the word "latex" on the package.

☐ Handle the condom carefully to avoid damaging it with fingernails, teeth, or other sharp objects.

☐ Always use a condom from start to finish: Put the condom on after the penis is erect and before any contact with the partner's vagina, mouth, or anus. (If the penis is uncircumcised, pull the foreskin back before putting on the condom.) After ejaculation, withdraw the penis while it is still erect, holding on to the rim of the condom so that it doesn't come off.

☐ Put the condom on by rolling it down over the penis. Never unroll the condom before putting it on.

☐ Leave a small space (a half inch) in the top of the condom to catch the semen, or use a condom with a reservoir tip. Pinch the tip before rolling the condom down over the penis so that no air is trapped. Remove any air that remains in the tip by gently pressing toward the base of the penis. Air in the tip can make the condom break.

☐ Lubrication on condoms may help prevent them from tearing during vaginal or anal sex. You can purchase prelubricated condoms, and/or add your own lubricant, which should be water-based (check the label). Lubricants containing the spermicide nonoxynol-9 offer additional protection against HIV, other STDs, and pregnancy. Do not use oil-based lubricants such as petroleum jelly, cold cream, baby oil, cooking oil, massage oil, or shortening. These weaken latex and can often cause the condom to break. Nonlubricated condoms are preferable for oral sex, and some are available in flavors like mint.

- If you feel the condom slip off or break while having sex, stop immediately. The penis should be withdrawn, and intercourse should not continue until a new condom is put on.

- Never use a condom more than once.

- Do not use condoms when their expiration date (written on the package) has passed, when their packaging is damaged, or when they show obvious signs of deterioration—such as brittleness, stickiness, or discoloration.

- Do not store condoms near heat and do not keep them in your wallet or a car's glove compartment for a long time. Instead, store condoms in a cool, dry place out of direct sunlight—a drawer or closet might be appropriate.

- To more safely perform oral sex on a woman, cut an unlubricated condom lengthwise down the middle and hold it so it covers her vulva (the entrance to the vagina). Microwavable plastic wrap (such as Saran Wrap) can be used the same way. When performing oral-anal sex, a plastic barrier is placed over the anus of the receptive partner. (Note: Plastic wrap is not an effective substitute for a condom for vaginal or anal intercourse.)

- It is not safe to practice "withdrawal," in which the man pulls his penis out of his partner's body before he ejaculates, as a substitute for condoms. Like semen, pre-ejaculatory fluid may contain HIV and transmit the virus.

- Using contraceptives other than condoms, including diaphragms and birth control pills, will protect you from pregnancy but not from HIV or other STDs.

alternative for people who are allergic to latex, the device offers these advantages: it is thinner than latex, has no odor, and can be used safely with oil-based lubricants.

Dealing With a Partner Who Won't Use Condoms. Although your partner may be glad and relieved when you say you want to use a condom, it is possible that he or she will reject the idea. Your lover may believe it is not necessary. Many people think they cannot have HIV because they are not ill. (They also might assume that the same is true of their partners.) But you do not need to have symptoms to harbor the AIDS virus—or to pass it on to someone else. Most teens with HIV are symptom free and do not know they have the virus. *You cannot tell from someone's appearance whether or not the person has HIV.*

Some people feel that condoms decrease the pleasure of sex or that they interfere with sexual performance. But with a little practice, this should not be a problem. Also, when you use condoms, both partners will feel less anxious about AIDS because both are protected. This can let you relax and enjoy being together.

Males are more likely to be the ones to resist a female's request to use a condom, rather than the other way around. Explain to your partner why you want to use a condom, and say that it is for his protection too. Showing him a book like this one, or a magazine article on AIDS and safer sex, may help convince him. If it does not, refusing to have intercourse is your safest and simplest option. You can still have worry-free outercourse if your partner agrees.

A decision to have intercourse without a condom should not be made lightly. You need to know for

No Condom? No Sex!

It might help to practice in advance what you would say to a person who resists using condoms. Some possibilities are:

☐ "I care for you but I cannot make love to you without a condom."

☐ "I love the way you touch me. If you don't want to use a condom, we can touch without having intercourse."

☐ "If you want to have sex without a condom, you'll have to do it without me."

Try to think of other things to say that seem natural to you. Women whose partners refuse condoms may decide to use the female condom.

certain that your partner is HIV-negative. Even if you have known someone a long time and trust him or her, it is no guarantee that the person does not have HIV. The closest you can come to being certain is to ask your partner to take an HIV test (see Chapter 6) and to accompany him or her to get the results. (It is also possible that your partner has another STD but is not aware of it. STDs such as herpes and genital warts may have no visible signs but still be infectious. A condom helps prevent transmission in this case.)

Second best is to know whether your partner is at increased risk for HIV infection because of his or her health history. A partner at increased risk will pose a greater danger to you. But even if your lover says he or she is not at high risk, it might make sense to ask yourself this question: If my partner doesn't want to use condoms with me, does that make it more likely condoms were not used with previous partners? You cannot know for sure that your partner is telling you the whole truth about his or her history—or that your partner will remain uninfected—so a condom is always your best bet.

Avoid High-Risk Partners

People are considered to be at increased risk for being infected with the AIDS virus if they have:

1. shared drug-injecting equipment

2. had unprotected sex with other males and they are male

3. had unprotected sex with someone they knew or suspected had HIV

4. had an STD

5. had unprotected sex with many different people

6. received a blood transfusion or blood products before 1985

7. had unprotected sex with anyone who has done anything in items 1-6

If your partner or partners are at increased risk for HIV, this will in turn make it more likely that you could become infected. In general, even if you are using condoms, it is safer to have partners at low risk.

Limiting How Many Partners You Have. You can decrease your risk of contracting HIV by limiting the number of people you have sex with. The fewer sexual partners you have, the lower your risk. Conversely, the more people you have sex with, the greater your risk.

Your safest option is to have intercourse only in a long-term relationship in which both you and your partner are HIV-negative and monogamous (meaning neither of you has sex with anyone else), and neither injects drugs. You should each understand that if either partner engages in any risky behavior outside the relationship, it could endanger both members of the couple.

Because people are often tempted to be unfaithful and do not always reveal when they cheat, it would still be more realistic, and safer, for teens to use condoms even in a monogamous relationship. But it may be difficult to use condoms in this kind of relationship because of the trust issue. For instance, a boy may wonder whether his girlfriend's insistence on using condoms means she does not trust him. A girl may wonder if her boyfriend uses condoms because he has been unfaithful.

There are no easy answers to this dilemma. In general though, it is not fair for your lover to refuse your request to use condoms. You should not have to risk your life unnecessarily to prove you trust someone. If your lover refuses condoms, you might want to consider alternatives to intercourse—or reconsider the relationship.

HIV and Drugs

HIV can also be transmitted when people who use injectable drugs—such as cocaine, heroin, and steroids—share their injecting equipment without cleaning it first. A person injects drugs using a

Are You At Risk?

The Relative Safety of Different Sex Acts

The Most Dangerous

Unprotected Anal Intercourse

Very Dangerous

Unprotected Vaginal Intercourse

Potentially Dangerous

Unprotected Oral Intercourse

Safer

Any Intercourse with a Latex Condom
(used correctly and every time)

Almost Completely Safe

Kissing, Hugging, Petting, Massage, Mutual
Masturbation, Licking (not including oral sex)

Completely Safe

Abstinence; Self-masturbation

syringe, a hollow plastic tube that holds the drugs. The syringe is fitted with a plunger at one end and a hollow needle at the other.

This is how two drug users—we will call them Alan and Susan—transmit HIV between themselves. Alan, who has HIV, sticks a hypodermic needle into his body— maybe directly into a vein, maybe under the skin. He depresses the plunger to "shoot" the drug through the needle and into his skin, muscle, or bloodstream. When he withdraws the needle, a few drops of his blood flow out of his body and up into the needle and syringe. Next, Susan uses the same equipment without cleaning it. Alan's infected blood mixes with Susan's drugs in the syringe. When she shoots up, she gets high . . . and she may get a dose of HIV right in her bloodstream.

Injecting drugs is dangerous. If you don't inject drugs, AIDS is a powerful additional reason not to start. If you do inject drugs, the safest course to take is to stop. If you quit, you will never have to worry about getting HIV from a needle. And if you give up all drugs, you will avoid their other hazards—possible arrest, addiction, overdose, and health problems. For help in quitting, call a local drug rehabilitation center. Look in the Yellow Pages under "Drug Abuse and Addiction—Information and Treatment."

If you inject drugs, you should never share needles or syringes with, or borrow them from, anyone else. You should not reuse needles either. Do not buy or rent such equipment on the street—in many cases it has been used, even if the seller claims it is new. Also, you should not reuse or share cotton balls, "cookers," rinse or wash water, or other equipment used in preparing and injecting drugs—these items may be contaminated with blood.

Some cities such as New York offer needle exchange programs (see Chapter 4) that let drug users get new needles legally, typically by trading in old ones. Call your local department of health to find out if such a program is available near you.

You may also be able to buy hypodermic needles at a drugstore, although laws in some states prohibit buying or owning them without a prescription. If you cannot get new needles or syringes, cleaning injection equipment properly will reduce the risk of HIV infection. There is only one way to do this: by using clean water, then bleach, which kills HIV.

Needles and syringes are made to be used only one time. Cleaning your equipment with bleach is not as safe as using a new, sterile needle and syringe. It will not ensure that you do not become infected, but it will significantly improve your chances of avoiding the AIDS virus. Follow the steps listed below and shown in the diagram:

DO STEPS 1-3 IN SEQUENCE THREE TIMES:

1. Dip needle into a cup of clean water (the water should first be boiled or be as hot as possible from the faucet), then draw water up into syringe.

2. Withdraw needle from water, then shake syringe several times.

3. Push out syringe contents into a sink or toilet. (Do not inject or drink the water.)

DO STEP 4 THREE TIMES:

4. Repeat steps 1 through 3, but instead of water use common household bleach, such as Clorox.

DO STEP 5 THREE TIMES:

5. Repeat steps 1 through 3, using water again.

How to Clean Needles

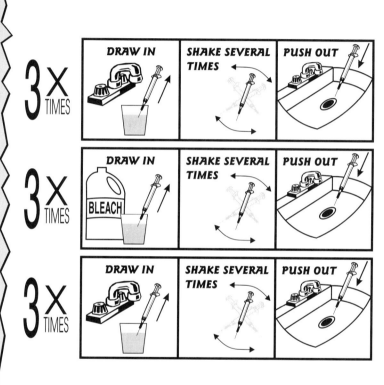

Other cleaning methods do not work. Boiling your equipment for a short time is not sufficient, nor is holding it over a match.

In addition to their other dangers, illegal drugs and alcohol can cloud your judgment about unsafe sexual behaviors. For instance, they may weaken your resolve to abstain from sex, to practice only outer-course, or to always use a condom. If you are very high or drunk, it could be more difficult to put on and take off a condom correctly. Also, it may be harder to communicate with your partner about safer sex. So you are better off staying sober; and if you are drunk or high, you are better off not having sex.

6

If You Are at Risk . . .

If your history does not put you at risk for HIV, you are unlikely to harbor the virus. But if you have any risk factors for HIV, you cannot know for sure if you are infected (and neither can your sex partners). If you are healthy, you may have HIV that has not yet caused any symptoms; if you are ill, it could be from another cause.

HIV Testing

The only way to be sure one way or another is to have your blood tested for the AIDS virus. Some people—for instance, those who have never injected illegal drugs, never had sex, and never received a blood transfusion—may have no need to get tested. But there are others who should consider this option seriously.

The Decision. People take the HIV test for several reasons. Some are at increased risk for having HIV (see page 78) or are sick, and want to know whether they are actually HIV infected. Some couples take the test before having intercourse—or before making their relationship exclusive—to be sure neither partner is infected. And other individuals are just anxious about AIDS and want to be absolutely certain about their HIV status.

In the following list are some reasons why you might want to get tested. If your test results are "negative," you are probably (but not necessarily, see page 91) HIV-negative and do not have the virus. This may be useful to know because:

▢ It may come as a relief. Despite any risks you may have taken in the past, you are not infected. Now, by learning to avoid those dangerous behaviors, you can make sure you do not become infected in the future.

▢ Counseling provided when you take the test should help you learn how to avoid future infection.

▢ Your doctor can rule out HIV as a cause of any illnesses you may have. This could help in diagnosis.

If your results are "positive," you are almost definitely infected. Having this information may help you too:

▢ Recent breakthroughs in drug treatment mean that for many people HIV infection is probably no longer a death sentence. Learning your HIV status and getting proper treatment from a doctor may very well prevent you from going on to develop AIDS.

◻ Your doctor will be able to determine the cause and best treatment of any diseases you may have now or in the future. Tuberculosis and syphilis, for instance, are treated differently in people who are HIV-positive and HIV-negative.

◻ Doctors can monitor your immune system, and if it weakens, they can prevent or more effectively treat AIDS-related illnesses. Vaccinations can protect you from common hazards like bacterial pneumonia and flu.

◻ You can make lifestyle changes that may keep you healthier, such as eating well, exercising, and avoiding drugs and alcohol.

◻ You will be able to make a better decision about whether to get pregnant or to continue a pregnancy. If you decide to have a baby, the drug AZT can greatly reduce the chances that your newborn will also be infected.

◻ You can take steps to help preserve other people's health. If your lover is uninfected, you can protect him or her by always using a condom or by abstaining from sex. You can warn former sex partners that they are potentially at risk and should also consider being tested.

◻ Counseling provided when you get an HIV test can tell you what your results mean, and what actions you should take now that you know them.

One problem with testing is the privacy issue. Although you might take the test anonymously or confidentially, you would probably want to inform your doctor, and possibly others, about a positive result. Eventually, someone may find out about your condition without your permission. Also, employers and health insurers may learn about your HIV status if it becomes part of your medical record. One result of people finding out you are infected could be discrimination—legal or illegal—at school, on the job, or in housing or insurance.

To learn more about HIV testing, talk to a counselor at a testing site or elsewhere. Although you may be reluctant to get tested, the new treatments available for people with the AIDS virus are an extremely powerful argument for doing so. If you are at risk and elect not to get tested, though, you should take measures to protect others. Since you *might* have the virus, don't have sex at all—or at least don't have unprotected sex—and don't share hypodermic needles.

The Procedure. HIV tests may be offered at family planning, STD, hospital, or community health clinics; publicly funded HIV testing centers; drug treatment facilities; and your doctor's office. Most places offer either confidential or anonymous testing. Depending on the state where you take the test, you may or may not need your parents' permission.

In confidential testing, your name and test result are recorded but not revealed to anyone except medical personnel and, in some states, the state health department. In anonymous testing, which is not available everywhere, you do not give your name. You use an assigned code to get your results, and no one else will learn them unless you decide to share the information.

To get information on where to go in your area for testing, call the Centers for Disease Control and Prevention National AIDS Hotline at 1-800-342-AIDS. Then call the testing site and make an appointment. Because the test is in great demand, you may have to wait a few weeks before they can see you.

Before your test, a counselor at the testing site should speak to you. He or she might ask questions to find out if testing is appropriate for you. If it is, the counselor should:

☐ give you information about AIDS, HIV, and its transmission

☐ explain the confidentiality of test results

☐ explain how you will be informed of the results

☐ discuss what the different possible test results mean

☐ answer any questions you may have (you might want to make a list ahead of time)

The medical procedure you go through when you get tested is very simple; you may have experienced it before when you went to the doctor for a checkup or to be treated for an illness. A health professional draws a small quantity of blood from your arm and then sends it to a laboratory. You will have to wait a few days or longer to get the results of tests carried out at the lab. During this period, protect sex and drug-using partners from the possibility that you do have HIV—don't have sex without a condom, or don't have sex at all, and don't share needles.

When any virus enters your body, your immune

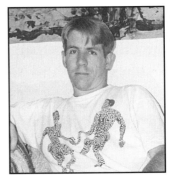

Kevin Irvine

Kevin Irvine, age twenty-six, a skills trainer and advocate for people with disabilities, lives in Albuquerque, New Mexico. Growing up with severe hemophilia in Palo Alto, California, Kevin was open about his condition until his teen years when the AIDS epidemic struck. Having no symptoms of HIV infection but fearing the stigma of AIDS, he stopped discussing his hemophilia. When he was sixteen years old a medical test confirmed his fears—he was HIV-positive.

For the next four years Kevin says he was "in denial" about the diagnosis and would not discuss it in depth with anyone. At the same time, the counseling he got was inadequate. "They told me about condoms, but not how to use them." Between his refusing to deal with the fact that he had HIV and his lack of skills in preventing its transmission, he was definitely not prepared for sexual activity. But he was, he says, a "hormone-addled adolescent" who very much wanted to have sex.

In his junior year at college Kevin took a class on AIDS, met others who were HIV-positive, and "realized there was a life beyond being sad and lonely about HIV." Eventually he decided to be open about having HIV and to educate other young people so they would not get it.

He has a powerful message for them: Although he knows now it was wrong, in high school he lied to get sex. "I didn't use condoms and I told two of my partners they had nothing to worry about. People lie all the time to get sex. Use condoms . . . your partners could be lying, or may not even know their HIV status."

Luckily, none of Kevin's partners contracted HIV. Kevin has had the AIDS virus for more than ten years and has never been sick from it. He now discloses his HIV status to the women he dates.

system responds by making proteins called antibodies that attack it. The body produces different antibodies in response to different viruses. The body responds to HIV infection by making antibodies to HIV. (As we learned in Chapter 2, attacks by these antibodies are unsuccessful in ridding the body of the virus.) An HIV test looks for these antibodies. If it finds them, that means you have been infected.

Lab workers use two types of HIV-antibody tests. The first, called ELISA (for "enzyme-linked immunosorbent assay"), is a screening test that can tell doctors only whether or not the presence of HIV antibodies is a possibility. If the ELISA test is positive (antibodies may be in the blood), another test called the Western blot is performed to confirm the results. Together, the two tests are more than 99.9 percent accurate.

The Results. If your test is negative, antibodies to HIV were not found in your blood. It is likely, then, that you do not have HIV. It is possible, however, that you are infected but the test failed to detect it. This could be the case if you recently engaged in behavior that can transmit HIV.

It can take a while—usually three months at most but, rarely, as long as six months—for your body to produce antibodies in response to HIV. So if you had unprotected sex or shared needles less than six months before the test, you could be infected but still test negative. To be sure, you must be tested again at least six months after any risky behavior.

If both the ELISA and Western blot tests are positive, you have almost definitely been infected with HIV. There is a tiny possibility that the result is a "false positive," which means no antibody was in your blood and the reading was in error. If this was your first positive test, you can eliminate this possibility by getting retested.

Whether your test is negative or positive, you should receive counseling again after you get the results. If you are HIV-negative, your counselor may review what you can do to stay that way. Just because you do not have HIV now, it does not mean you cannot get it in the future. Anyone can contract the virus anytime he or she does something risky. So you still should follow the rules about safe behavior. (However, that does not mean you cannot be friends with people who have HIV or AIDS. Such people may need your help and support, and you will not become infected by offering hugs or running errands.)

If your test was positive, your counselor should discuss what this means for you. He or she will also answer your questions; refer you for follow-up health care, support services, or further counseling; and talk to you about informing your lovers or needle-sharing partners.

If You Have HIV . . .

A positive test result means only that you have been infected, not necessarily that you have AIDS. Most people who are infected do not have AIDS, although if they are not treated, they are likely to develop it eventually. The test cannot tell when this will happen. Half of untreated people with HIV do not get AIDS for at least ten years. They may be perfectly healthy or only mildly ill until then.

Getting prompt medical attention will improve your odds in the fight against HIV infection: new drugs, discussed in Chapter 2, may prevent the onset of AIDS and save your life. So if your test was positive, make an appointment with a doctor, even if you are feeling fine. Let your physician know you have HIV. He or she should be familiar with HIV/AIDS treatment or refer you to another doctor who is. Your physician should do a complete checkup, as well as a blood test to check your T cell count. This test will show how well your immune system is functioning. Be sure to follow your doctor's instructions and take prescribed drugs regularly.

If you have been infected, you can pass the virus to another person, who in turn may transmit it to someone else, and so on. You can help stop this train of events by taking the following measures:

▢ Never have unprotected sex or share drug-injecting equipment.

(Do not assume that a sex partner willing to have unsafe sex is HIV-positive also; it is just as likely that the person does not have HIV but, for whatever reasons, won't take precautions.) In addition to protecting your partner from HIV and other STDs, using a condom protects you—by reducing your chances of getting another sexually transmitted disease. STDs may be more difficult to cure in people with HIV and can also bring on AIDS faster.

▢ Young women with HIV should understand the risks of pregnancy. The virus can be transmitted to the fetus while in the uterus, during childbirth, or during breastfeeding. If you receive the drug AZT during your pregnancy and labor, the chances of transmission to the baby are reduced from one out of four to

Protect Your Health

Here are some other steps you should take to protect your health if you are HIV-positive:

☐ Get tested for tuberculosis (TB). You could be infected with the bacteria that causes this disease and not know it. If you have TB and it is not discovered, it could make you seriously ill. However, if found early in HIV infection, TB can be treated successfully.

☐ Vaccines for flu and other infections may protect your health by preventing disease. Ask your doctor about getting vaccinated.

☐ Tell your doctor if you get any of the following symptoms, which may be linked to HIV:

—swollen glands in the neck, armpits, or groin

—white patches in your mouth

—bruises or sores on your skin that don't heal

—fever or diarrhea

—failure to gain weight, if you are still growing; or weight loss, if you have stopped growing

—coughing or shortness of breath

—night sweats

—severe headaches

—vaginal yeast infections that do not clear up when treated

—irregular menstrual bleeding, or persistent pain in the abdomen

☐ Eat a healthy diet. Get advice on this from a doctor or nurse.

- Get plenty of rest; avoid stress and exhausting activities. Make time to do things you enjoy.

- Do some form of exercise that you like. Exercise will not only make you stronger, it will also help combat stress.

- Recreational drugs, tobacco, and heavy use of alcohol can all weaken your body and make it more difficult to fight off disease. If you use any of these substances, it is best to stop. If you find this too difficult, consider enrolling in a program designed to help you quit.

- New drugs for treating HIV or diseases associated with it are tested in clinical trials, in which volunteers take the medicines to see if they work. If the test is successful, you may have a new tool to improve your health. The information gained during such experimental trials may help other people as well. Ask your doctor or clinic if any trials are being held in your area, or call the AIDS Clinical Trials Information Service (1-800-TRIALS-A).

- You might want to join a support group for people who are HIV-positive if one is available in your area. Such a group could give you emotional support and practical help in dealing with HIV infection. Find out about groups in your area by asking your doctor or calling your local health department.

- Get as much support as possible from family and friends. You can accept offers of help, be near them, and enjoy their hugs and kisses without worry—HIV cannot be transmitted by any of these activities.

one out of twelve. The baby must receive AZT for several weeks after birth and should not be breast-fed by the infected mother.

☐ Because your body tissues and organs could carry HIV, you should not donate them, whether during your life or after your death. This means you should not donate blood, organs, sperm, eyes, or bone marrow. Do not sign a form permitting organ donation upon your death, and withdraw any such permission you might have given already.

☐ If your blood, from a cut or nosebleed, spills on clothing, furniture, or other surfaces, clean it off as follows: (1) Use soap and water. (2) Clean again with a disinfectant, alcohol, or a mixture of one part household bleach and nine parts water. (3) Wash your hands with soap and water. You can use the same procedure for cleaning off semen and saliva.

☐ Do not share a razor, or any other item that may touch your blood, semen, or vaginal fluids, with someone else.

☐ Inform any physician or dentist who provides you with medical care that you have HIV.

☐ Reveal your test results to any of your partners—especially current or recent ones—with whom you have had unprotected sex or shared drug-injecting equipment. Explain that they may be infected and need to be counseled and tested. Your own testing counselor or other health care professional can inform these people for you (without revealing your name) or help you do it yourself. It is important that your partners be notified quickly, as this will allow them to get prompt medical care and make it less likely that they will infect others. Informing current or former partners can be emotionally difficult. If you do it yourself, do not accuse them. Be ready for them to become hostile or distressed.

Keep in mind that if you feel comfortable telling friends or others you have the AIDS virus, you may help them by doing so. Many young people do not believe they could actually become infected with HIV. But their view sometimes changes when they know someone who is HIV-positive because it makes the threat seem more real. Then it is more likely that they will take steps to reduce their risk and that, if necessary, they will get tested for HIV themselves.

Where to Find Help

Hotlines

National AIDS Hotline

1-800-342-2437

Answers any questions on HIV and AIDS, gives referrals to HIV-testing and counseling sites, and provides information about AIDS prevention and treatment. Operates twenty-four hours a day.

National STD Hotline

1-800-227-8922

Answers questions on prevention and treatment of all sexually transmitted diseases. Operates 8:00 A.M. to 11:00 P.M., Eastern Standard Time, Monday to Friday.

AIDS Clinical Trials Information Service

1-800-TRIALS-A

Provides information on trials of experimental drugs for treating HIV or diseases associated with it. Operates 9:00 A.M. to 7:00 P.M., Eastern Standard Time, Monday to Friday.

1-800-ALCOHOL

Makes referrals to facilities that provide treatment for drug and alcohol addiction. Also makes referrals to twelve-step programs aimed at dealing with addiction. Operates twenty-four hours a day.

Teens Teaching AIDS Prevention

1-800-234-TEEN

Trained teens age thirteen to twenty answer questions on HIV testing, sex, AIDS, and related topics, and make referrals to local hotlines across the country. Operates 4:00 P.M. to 8:00 P.M., Central Standard Time, Monday to Friday.

National Runaway Switchboard

1-800-621-4000

Helps adolescents in crisis sort out their options, and get the resources they need to deal with any problem, including questions about HIV and AIDS. Makes referrals. Operates twenty-four hours a day throughout the year.

Project Inform

1-800-822-7422

This organization provides comprehensive information on treatment for HIV/AIDS, including clinical trials of new drugs, nutrition, and alternative medicine. Operates 10:00 A.M. to 4:00 P.M., Pacific Standard Time, Monday to Saturday.

Chapter Notes

Chapter 1

1. Centers for Disease Control and Prevention, *HIV/AIDS Surveillance Report*, Atlanta, 1995, vol. 7, no. 1, pp. 8, 14.

2. Gabriel Torres, "Second National Retrovirus Conference," *GMHC Treatment Issues* (newsletter of Gay Men's Health Crisis), March 1995, p. 4.

3. Associated Press, "WHO Starts Hunt for HIV Barrier," *The New York Times*, November 17, 1993, p. C17.

4. Donatella Lorch, "After Years of Ignoring AIDS Epidemic, Kenya Has Begun Facing Up to It," *The New York Times*, December 18, 1993, p. 5; and "Rapid Rise of AIDS in Asia Aggravating Risk of Tuberculosis," *The New York Times*, August 11, 1994, p. A16.

5. Randy Kennedy, "Neighborhood Report: West Village," *The New York Times*, June 19, 1994, sec. 14, p. 6.

6. Jane Gross, "Second Wave of AIDS Feared by Officials in San Francisco," *The New York Times*, December 11, 1993, p. 1.

7. Abraham Verghese, *My Own Country: A Doctor's Story* (New York: Vintage Books, 1995); also, Perri Klass, "AIDS in the Heartland" (book review), *The New York Times*, August 28, 1994, sec. 7, p. 1.

8. "The Changing Face of AIDS" (editorial), *New York Newsday*, April 9, 1995, pp. A21–A22.

9. Felicia R. Lee, "On a Harlem Block, Hope Is Swallowed by Decay," *The New York Times*, September 8, 1994, p. A1.

10. Reuters, "Blacks Far More Likely Than Whites to Have AIDS, Agency Says," *The New York Times*, September 9, 1994, p. A16.

11. Ibid.

12. Felicia R. Lee, "Federal Cuts Set Off Debate on Homeless with AIDS," *The New York Times*, March 21, 1995, p. B1.

13. Centers for Disease Control and U.S. Department of Health and Human Services, *Morbidity and Mortality Weekly Report*, February 10, 1995, vol. 44, no. 5, p. 81.

14. Felicia R. Lee, "Anguish in Era of AIDS: Choosing to Have Babies," *The New York Times*, May 9, 1995, p. A1.

15. Joanne Wasserman, "Moms with AIDS File Memories for Their Kids," *Daily News*, February 9, 1995, p. 54.

Chapter 2

1. Abraham Verghese, *My Own Country: A Doctor's Story* (New York: Vintage Books, 1995), p. 102.

2. U.S. Department of Health and Human Services, Agency for Health Care Policy and Research, *HIV and Your Child* (AHCPR Pub. No. 94-0576), January 1994, p. 2.

3. Both cases referred to in this paragraph are discussed in Lawrence K. Altman, "AIDS Mystery That Won't Go Away," *The New York Times*, July 5, 1994, p. C3; and Reuters, "AIDS Claims 4th Patient of Florida Dentist," *The New York Times*, December 19, 1994, p. A14.

4. Lawrence K. Altman, "In 2 Young Patients, Rare Transmission of HIV Is Detected," *The New York Times*, December 4, 1993, p. 1.

5. Lawrence K. Altman, "Scientists Report Unusual Transmissions of H.I.V.," *The New York Times*, December 5, 1993, p. 32.

6. John L. Ingraham and Catherine A. Ingraham, *Introduction to Microbiology* (Belmont, Calif.: Wadsworth, 1995), p. 542.

7. Mireya Navarro, "Confining Tuberculosis Patients," *The New York Times*, November 21, 1993, p. A1.

8. Lawrence K. Altman, "In Major Finding, Drug Curbs H.I.V. Infection in Newborns," *The New York Times*, February 21, 1994, p. A1.

9. Christine Gorman, "The Exorcists," *Time*, special issue, "The Frontiers of Medicine," Fall 1996, pp. 64–65.

10. Gina Kolata, "New Studies Offer Powerful and Puzzling Evidence on Immunity to AIDS," *The New York Times*, September 27, 1996, p. A27.

11. Jesse Green, "Who Put the Lid on gp120?" *The New York Times Sunday Magazine*, March 26, 1995, sec. 6, p. 50ff.

12. Isabelle de Vincenzi, M.D., "A Longitudinal Study of Human Immunodeficiency Virus Transmission by Heterosexual Partners," *New England Journal of Medicine*, August 11, 1994, p. 341.

Other Sources:

Michael Thomas Ford, *100 Questions and Answers About AIDS* (New York: Beech Tree Books, 1993).

Karen Hein and Theresa Foy DiGeronimo, *AIDS: Trading Fears for Facts*, 3rd ed. (Yonkers, N.Y.: Consumer Reports, 1993).

Daniel Jussim, *Medical Ethics: Moral and Legal Conflicts in Health Care* (Englewood Cliffs, N.J.: Julian Messner, 1991).

Alvin and Virginia Silverstein, *AIDS: Deadly Threat* (Hillside, N.J.: Enslow Publishers, Inc., 1991).

Chapter 3

1. The material on Ryan White is from David Kirp, *Learning by Heart: AIDS and Schoolchildren in America's Communities* (New Brunswick, N.J.: Rutgers University Press, 1989), pp. 26–64; Ann Marie Cunningham, "I Don't Want My Son to Be Forgotten," *Ladies Home Journal*, August 1990, p. 102ff; and Mary Kittredge, *Teens with AIDS Speak Out* (Englewood Cliffs, N.J.: Julian Messner, 1991), pp. 50–52.

2. Centers for Disease Control and Prevention, *HIV/AIDS Surveillance Report*, Atlanta, 1995, vol. 7, no. 1, pp. 8, 12.

3. Cunningham, p. 161.

4. Kirp, p. 36.

5. Quoted in Abraham Verghese, *My Own Country: A Doctor's Story* (New York: Vintage, 1995), p. 160.

6. The story of Mark Hoyle is discussed in Kirp, pp. 65–93.

7. Mireya Navarro, "Children with a Secret (Spelled AIDS)," *The New York Times*, March 28, 1991, p. A1.

8. His story is told in Michael T. Kaufman, "A Hero in the AIDS Battle and a Fun-Loving Boy," *The New York Times*, November 24, 1993, p. B3; and in Navarro, p. A1.

Chapter 4

1. John J. O'Connor, "Young People Confronting AIDS," *The New York Times*, June 6, 1995.

2. Edward McCabe, "Our 'Just Say No' School Board," *The New York Times*, May 30, 1994, p. 15.

3. National Commission on AIDS, *Preventing HIV/AIDS in Adolescents*, Washington, D.C., 1993, p. 3.

4. Linda Saslow, "Teen-agers Educate Teen-agers about Realities of AIDS," *The New York Times*, April 24, 1994, sec. 14LI, p. 12.

5. Ibid.

6. Statistics in this paragraph are from Centers for Disease Control and Prevention, *HIV/AIDS Surveillance Report*, Atlanta, 1995, vol. 7, no. 1, pp. 12–13. The numbers reflect total cumulative AIDS cases reported through June 1995.

7. Joseph F. Sullivan, "Assembly Again Passes Sexual-Abstinence Bill," *The New York Times*, December 2, 1994, p. B5.

8. Sam Dillon, "AIDS Council to Review Guide for High Schools," *The New York Times*, October 22, 1994, p. 27.

9. As discussed in Barbara Defoe Whitehead, "The Failure of Sex Education," *The Atlantic Monthly*, October 1994, pp. 55–80.

10. Heather J. Walter and Roger D. Vaughan, "AIDS Risk Reduction Among a Multiethnic Sample of Urban High School Students," *Journal of the American Medical Association*, August 11, 1993, p. 725.

11. Quoted in Jane Gross, "Second Wave of AIDS Feared by Officials in San Francisco," *The New York Times*, December 11, 1993, p. 1.

12. Saslow, sec. 14LI, p. 12.

13. National Commission on AIDS, p. 13.

14. Saslow, sec. 14LI, p. 12.

15. Josh Barbanel, "Condom Handouts Voided in Schools," *The New York Times*, December 31, 1993, p. A1.

16. McCabe, p. 15.

17. Christopher Wiss, "Preventing AIDS in the 90s," *The Volunteer* (GMHC newsletter), March/April 1995, pp. 5–6.

18. Felicia R. Lee, "Needle Exchange Program Shown to Slow H.I.V. Rates," *The New York Times*, November 26, 1994, p. 1.

19. "Clean Needles Slow AIDS" (editorial), *The New York Times*, December 6, 1994, p. A22.

20. Associated Press, "Citizen Arrests Challenge Needle Exchanges," *The New York Times*, September 18, 1994, p. 38; and Associated Press, "Needle Exchanges Backed," *The New York Times*, September 8, 1994, p. A16.

21. Nancy Sosman, "Needle Exchanges Destroy Neighborhoods," letter to the editor, *The New York Times*, December 6, 1994, p. A22.

22. Gross, p. 1.

23. Philip J. Hilts, "Lack of Studies on Sex Limits AIDS Research," *The New York Times*, July 28, 1994, p. A18.

Glossary

abstinence—Refraining from doing something, such as having sex.

AIDS—The acronym for acquired immunodeficiency syndrome, a deadly disease in which a person's immune system is weakened, making him or her vulnerable to unusual cancers and infections.

anal intercourse—A sex act in which a man inserts his penis into his partner's rectum, via the anus.

AZT (azidothymidine)—An antiviral drug used to slow the growth of HIV. It blocks the enzyme known as reverse transcriptase, which HIV needs to reproduce.

blood transfusion—The introduction of prepared blood, often donated by a different person, into someone's body (such as during surgery or after an accident).

condom—A sheath worn over the penis during intercourse. Latex condoms prevent pregnancy and sexually transmitted diseases, including AIDS.

epidemic—A disease affecting a large part of a population.

factor VIII—The protein in blood that lets it clot. Most hemophiliacs inject factor VIII concentrate, which is produced from donated blood, so their own blood can clot.

hemophiliac—A person with an inherited disease, which almost exclusively affects males, that prevents blood from clotting normally.

heterosexual intercourse—Sexual intercourse in which one person is male and the other female.

HIV—The abbreviation for human immunodeficiency virus, the virus that causes AIDS.

HIV-negative—Not infected with the AIDS virus.

HIV-positive—Infected with the AIDS virus.

homosexual intercourse—Sexual intercourse in which both people are male or both are female.

immune system—The bodily system that defends a person against harmful substances and germs.

injecting-drug user—A person who injects drugs, such as cocaine or heroin, using a hypodermic needle.

monogamous—Having a sexual relationship with only one partner.

oral intercourse—A sex act involving contact between one person's mouth and another person's penis, vagina, or anus.

pandemic—A disease affecting an unusually large percentage of people and occurring over a wide geographic area.

penis—The male sex organ and the channel through which a man's urine and semen pass.

pneumocystis pneumonia—A type of pneumonia caused by a common germ in people whose immune systems have been weakened, such as those with AIDS. The leading cause of death among AIDS patients.

protease inhibitors—A new family of antiviral drugs that fight HIV by blocking the enzyme known as protease, which the AIDS virus uses to reproduce.

rectum—The end of the intestines through which bowel movements, or stools, pass. This body part is penetrated by the partner's penis during anal intercourse.

retrovirus—A virus, such as HIV, that reverses the normal process by which a cell makes hereditary material and protein.

safer sex—A sex act in which precautions, such as the use of a condom during intercourse, are taken to minimize the risk of HIV transmission.

semen—The sperm-carrying fluid that is ejaculated by a man during sexual intercourse. If the man is infected with HIV, his semen may carry the virus and transmit it.

STD—The abbreviation for sexually transmitted disease, which can mean any disease, including AIDS, that is passed from one person to another during sexual intercourse.

T cell—A cell that plays an important role in coordinating the immune system's response to a harmful substance or invading germ. The depletion of T cells caused by HIV makes the body susceptible to cancers and infections that would normally be fought off easily.

tuberculosis (TB)—A communicable disease of the lungs caused by a bacterium. AIDS is partly responsible for the resurgence of TB in the United States.

unprotected intercourse—Intercourse without a latex condom.

vagina—A canal in the female that extends from the uterus to the outside of the body. This body part is penetrated by the penis during vaginal intercourse.

vaginal fluid—Lubricating liquid produced in the vagina that can carry and transmit HIV if the woman is infected.

vaginal intercourse—A sex act in which a man inserts his penis into a woman's vagina.

virus—an infection-causing agent that can reproduce only in the living cells of a plant or animal. It may be thought of as a simple life form or an extremely complex molecule.

Index

A

abstinence, 107
  debate over emphasis on in
    AIDS prevention
    programs, 52–58
  to prevent transmission of
    HIV, 67–69, 87
Africa, 6
African Americans, 13–15, 17,
    57, 71. *See also* minorities.
AIDS. *See also* HIV.
  as an epidemic, 8, 9
  definition of, 28, 107
  diseases associated with, 7,
    25–28
  geographical areas affected
    by, 8, 9, 12, 13
  groups most affected by,
    10–18
  history of, 6–8
  and homelessness, 16
  irrational fear of, 39–40
  number of people suffering
    from, 8, 9, 22, 36, 50, 51
  orphans created by, 17–18
  prevention programs, 48–65
    peer education, 58–59
    school-based, 50–60
      studies on, 56–58
  and schoolchildren, 34–47
  and social stigma, 40
  supporting people with, 47,
    92, 95
  treatments for, 29, 31, 32, 86,
    87, 93, 95
    expense of, 31, 32
  vaccines to prevent, 32–33
AIDS virus. *See* HIV.
anal intercourse, 21, 66, 67, 107

antibodies, 20, 91
anus, 67, 74
AZT (azidothymidine), 23, 29,
    43, 87, 93, 107

C

cancer, AIDS related, 7, 26. *See
    also* Kaposi's sarcoma.
Centers for Disease Control and
    Prevention, 27, 48, 49, 69
  National AIDS Hotline, 89
Clinton, Bill, 52, 62, 65
condoms, 7, 11, 12, 21, 33, 44,
    52, 53, 54, 58, 59, 60, 62, 67,
    68, 71, 72, 87, 89, 90, 93,
    107
  how to use, 72–76
  lubricated, 74
  made of polyurethane, 73, 76
  people who won't use, 7–8,
    11–12, 33, 76–78, 93
  programs to make available
    in schools, 52, 55, 59–60
  for women, 73, 77
conservatives, opinions on
    AIDS and sex education,
    52–53, 55–56

D

Danford, Alex, 5, 62
developing countries, 10, 31
DiPaolo, Joey, 45–47
drugs
  clinical trials of to treat
    HIV/AIDS, 5, 62, 95
  injection of and HIV
    transmission. *See* HIV,
    transmission of, through
    injection of illegal drugs.
  and risky sex, 61, 84

E
ejaculation, 67, 74, 75

F
factor VIII, 35, 36, 41, 107

G
gay men, 7, 10–13, 64–65
Gay Men's Health Crisis, 47, 61
genitals, 67
gonorrhea, 67
Goodlette, Pam, 5, 44
gp 120, 32–33

H
Hartley, Jody Lee, 6, 30
hemophilia, 5, 7, 23, 35, 36, 41,
    44, 90, 107
herpes, 49, 67, 77
heterosexual intercourse, 8, 21,
    66, 107
Hispanics, 13, 15, 17, 57. *See
    also* minorities.
HIV, 108. *See also* AIDS.
    rate of infection among
        teens, 50
    reproduction of inside
        human cells, 19, 28
    right of infected students to
        attend school, 37–38, 42
    in schoolchildren, 34–47
        parents keeping a secret,
            43, 45
    symptoms of infection by,
        25–26, 76, 94
    tests for the presence of, 23,
        44, 62, 77, 85–93
        anonymous, 88
        confidential, 88
        results of, 86, 91–93, 96
    transmission of, 20–25
        through accidents in
            health care setting, 24
        to babies from infected
            mothers, 7, 13, 21, 22,
            29, 87, 93, 96
        through blood
            transfusions or blood
            products, 5, 6, 7, 21, 22,

23, 35, 36, 41, 45, 51
        through casual contact,
            24–25, 37–42, 46
        through injection of
            illegal drugs, 7, 13, 14,
            21, 22, 47, 50, 51, 61,
            63, 64, 79, 81–84
        through sexual activity, 5,
            6, 7, 13, 14, 21, 22, 30,
            44, 47, 50, 51, 61, 62,
            66, 67, 69, 70, 71, 72,
            75, 80, 87, 93
        See also anal intercourse;
            heterosexual intercourse;
            homosexual intercourse;
            oral sex; vaginal
            intercourse.
homosexual intercourse, 8, 21,
    66, 108
homosexuality, 52, 53
homosexuals. *See* gay men.
Hoyle, Mark, 41, 42
human immunodeficiency
    virus. *See* HIV.

I
immune system, 7, 19–20, 62,
    87, 93, 108
Irvine, Kevin, 5, 90

K
Kaposi's sarcoma (KS), 26
Kirp, David, 39
kissing, 70, 95

L
liberals, opinions on AIDS and
    sex education, 52–54, 55
Lynch, Lisa, 6, 71

M
massage, 70
masturbation, 52, 70
    mutual, 70
minorities, 13–16. *See also*
    African Americans;
    Hispanics.
mouth, 70, 74

N

National Institutes of Health, 25
needles, hypodermic, 81, 82
    cleaning, 82–84
    exchange programs providing
        clean, 61, 63–64, 82
nonoxynol-9, 74

O

opportunistic infections, 26
oral sex, 66, 67, 75, 108
outercourse, 70, 76

P

penis, 67, 74, 75, 108
petting, 70
pneumocystis pneumonia, 26,
    32, 108
poverty, 13–16
pre-ejaculatory fluid, 67
protease inhibitors, 29, 31, 108

R

rectum, 67, 108

S

semen, 7, 21, 67, 96, 108
sex. See also sexual intercourse.
    with high-risk partners, 52,
        58, 77, 78
    limiting number of partners,
        79
    refusing, 56–58, 68–69
    safer, 8, 11, 12, 68, 69, 72, 76,
        80, 108
        debate over emphasis on
            in AIDS prevention
            programs, 52–61
    and trust issue, 71, 79
    and transmission of HIV. See
        HIV, transmission of,
        through sexual activity.
sexual abuse, 30

sexual intercourse, 74–75. See
    also anal intercourse;
    heterosexual intercourse;
    homosexual intercourse;
    oral sex; sex; vaginal
    intercourse.
sexually transmitted diseases.
    See STDS.
sperm. See semen.
STDs, 49, 53, 54, 67, 68, 74, 75,
    93, 109
support groups for people with
    AIDS, 61, 95
syphilis, 49, 67, 86
syringe, 81

T

T cells, 20, 26, 27, 28, 93, 109
teens,
    and ignorance about sex and
        consequences, 49, 50
    sexual behavior of, 48–50, 52,
        57
tuberculosis (TB), 27–28, 86, 94,
    109

U

United States, 6, 10, 27

V

vaccine,
    for AIDS, 5, 7
    for pneumonia and flu, 87,
        94
vagina, 67, 74, 109
vaginal fluid, 7, 21, 67, 96, 109
vaginal intercourse, 66, 109
viruses, definition of, 19, 109.
    See also HIV.

W

warts, genital, 77
White, Ryan, 35–40, 43
whites, 14, 15
women, 16–18, 50
World Health Organization, 10